How to
IMPROVE YOUR VISION

Robert A. Kraskin, O.D., F.A.A.O.

1976 EDITION

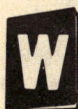

Published by
Melvin Powers
WILSHIRE BOOK COMPANY
12015 Sherman Road
No. Hollywood, California 91605
Telephone: (213) 875-1711

Printed by
HAL LEIGHTON PRINTING CO.
P.O. Box 1231
Beverly Hills, California 90213
Telephone: (213) 983-1105

Acknowledgments

Most of what I have come to believe about vision is the product of facts and ideas assimilated through years of contact with colleagues and patients.

Even though I cannot hope to name each of the persons who have had great influence on this book, the special contributions of a few must be specifically recognized. I should first mention the late Lewis H. Kraskin, O.D., not only because he was my father, but because he was also one of the pioneers of modern vision care. Although he lived only a year after my graduation from the Pennsylvania College of Optometry, my recollection of his determined research in the field of visual training did much to decide the direction of my interest.

Three other men stand out in my mind as professional fathers, because their friendship and counsel have influenced my approach to the practice of optometry. Moreover, they have been the leaders of a program that gives optometrists a unique opportunity to keep enlarging and updating their knowledge. These men are: Dr. E. B. Alexander, President of the Optometric Extension Program Foundation; Dr. Ralph Barstow, Director of

Optometric Professional Counselling for that Foundation; and Dr. A. M. Skeffington, the Foundation's Director of Education.

You will find the work of Darell Boyd Harmon, Ph.D., mentioned in later pages. Dr. Harmon is not an optometrist but an "educational scientist," specializing in ways to create a better learning environment for our students. His contributions to our profession and to the public welfare are countless.

In this book, as in my practice, I recognize that the patient is a full partner in every achievement. A doctor should always be learning, as well as teaching. The questions that my patients raise and the solutions we work out together underlie much of the progress that is being made. Some of these patients have become so convinced of the benefits of visual training that they have wished to work in my office as optometric assistants in order to help others. One of these merits particular mention, not so much because of her national prominence as because of her great dedication to visual care. As a worker in my office and as a public advocate, Miss Luci Johnson (now Mrs. Patrick Nugent) has never lost an opportunity to make others aware of what good vision means in their lives.

My sons Stephen and Jeffrey have had a special role in the development of the principles described in this book. To deal with visiting patients is one thing; to watch the visual development of one's own sons is even more convincing. I feel a little extra confidence in the advice I give to parents because of my experience with my own boys, beginning in their infancy and continuing into these years when they take an active interest in the observations that we make together.

The most important acknowledgment must go to my wife, whose contribution goes far beyond the patience and understanding required of any doctor's wife. She has always been first assistant in my office, as deeply involved as I am in vision care, a steady inspiration and a full-time co-worker. It is to my wonderful wife, Marion, that I dedicate this book.

Robert A. Kraskin, O.D.

Contents

INTRODUCTION

What This Book Will Do for You

The purpose of this book is to say in one short volume what I would like to be able to tell every patient and his family. There is so much that individuals can do for their own vision and that parents can do for their children's—apart from any professional help they may get. We all accept the fact that good or bad habits can contribute to body health or oral hygiene; your vision can be even more affected by your environment—home, school, office, or playground. I will try to suggest simple, practical ways to control environment so that you and your family will move in the direction of improved vision, rather than being resigned to the old idea of steady decline.

This book will also acquaint you with the greatest recent advance in the field of health care—one that can play a decisive role in your life.

During the past two generations, the combined efforts of many sciences have given us a new understanding of what vision is—going far beyond "eyesight" alone. The old optical theory of vision was "sight—with man left out" —as though the human body attached to a pair of eyes was incidental. That attitude persisted even after human behavior and the nervous system had begun to be explored in depth. But at last, with the help of experimental psychology, neurology, child development, cybernetics, and many other areas of science, a new dynamic approach to seeing was developed.

Vision, in the words of one pioneer, is the result of a very simple eye and a most complex brain. If it occurs mainly in the brain, then it affects the way we think—and the way we think can affect our vision.

Dr. Arnold Gesell braved a path by asserting: "To know the child, we must understand the nature of his vision." This led to the realization that what is true of the child is true at all ages—that vision is the dominant process of the whole human being.

World War II was one of the most important spurs to activity in this field, as in so many others. Many men were faced with the need for better vision in order to join a specific branch of the armed forces, and *visual-training* methods were developed to help them. In some of the services themselves, the need for greater perceptual efficiency—such as the ability to identify "friend" or "foe" in a split second—brought pressure for new methods. Since the war, the expanded interest in education, in career development, and even in avocations and sports, has put still greater demands on the visual system.

So, under the pressure of events, theory has been turned into fact. Viewing the human being as a total entity has made it possible to improve vision and many of the other body functions that are guided by vision.

A new profession has even grown up in response to the public need and demand for this new approach—optometry. Joining medicine and dentistry as a third major profession dealing with health, optometry now requires the same six-year college education, but the training is specifically directed to this over-all approach to vision care. In each state, the optometrist is the professional man specifically licensed to provide vision care and to recognize diseases of the eye. Whenever disease is found or medical treatment is needed, he refers the patient to an ophthalmologist, that is, a medical doctor who specializes in the eyes. Fortunately, it is relatively rare for the eyes themselves to be diseased or unhealthy, so the great majority of problems is based on *malfunction*. That's why there is a growing number of optometrists in the United States—about four times as many as ophthalmologists—and more of these are turning from the former role of mainly prescribing corrective lenses to the over-all approach to vision. Many optometrists, in fact, are taking continued postgraduate education in order to keep up with the flow of new knowledge.

The emphasis has changed from simple correction to prevention—and even to enhancement. In my own office, patients of all ages are told that there are three alternatives in vision care, depending on the individual's needs and desires:

1. Conventional care—which is usually a simple correction of problems in acuity (sharpness of eyesight).
2. Preventive care—to head off any problem that might

be threatening or to keep an existing one from getting worse.

3. Enhanced visual ability.

That last category can mean more ability in almost every other aspect of life as well—greater reading skill, an actual increase in IQ and all school or work performance, better physical co-ordination, more success in sports, more grace of bearing, a more relaxed and attractive personality.

All of these approaches will be described briefly in the chapters that follow, and I will also discuss the subject of seeing without glasses that has stirred so much controversy from time to time. Let me just say here that getting rid of eyeglasses is possible for some patients, but not for all. We now know that most visual problems result from childhood stresses—adaptations to some part of the child's very early environment or the stress of study later on. As some of these adaptations become so much a part of the individual's personality, it is often impractical to reverse them so completely that all lenses can be forgotten.

The over-all approach to maximum vision includes the use of lenses and visual training in many cases. This will often lessen or eliminate dependence on glasses for distance vision. What is of first importance is that it can guide the whole mental and neuromuscular make-up toward relaxed, first-class performance.

All the leading modern thoughts that have proven merit will be touched on in the pages to come. This is not intended to be the last word in visual care. New information will come with each passing year. But for you, this first realization of vision's role in your life can be the great breakthrough. You will find that insight into your visual system and how it relates to your entire body will be a major influence on your everyday activities.

CHAPTER 1

Vision Means Everything

The questions in your mind as you start this book are probably much like the ones that patients have always had when they have gone into an eye doctor's office—the ones I have spotlighted in the table of contents. I will touch on all of these and a good many others.

But today the answers are different, more advanced, more positive and hopeful. I can respond with more assurance than my own father could in the days when he was one of the pioneers of visual training. This kind of care has made long strides in the last two generations—some of the greatest in the whole field of human well-being. There have been discoveries of new facts about the eye, the retina, the neurological channels that connect with the brain. Laboratory researchers have given us some new pieces of hard information to use in helping people. But the greatest breakthrough has been due to a new conviction that most conditions formerly thought to be hereditary and beyond help need not be accepted with resignation. Just knowing that a problem is of our own making, rather than an inborn trait, is the first step toward finding a way out of it.

As we look together at the various ways of protecting your family's vision and of attacking any problems that may now exist, I want you to keep just a few key points firmly in mind:

- Vision is primarily in the brain, not in the eyes. *It is a conclusion reached by the brain* on the basis of data contributed by all the senses.
- The eyes are the organs that accept light, and therefore the most important source of the brain's information.
- But every other part of your body is also involved— from head to toe. The messages sent to the brain by your senses of touch, smell, taste, hearing, and balance all go to make up the final assessment of an object or a scene.
- Visual ability develops in a multitude of different ways—each person's way of seeing being a little different from anyone else's. This is due to the innumerable different stimuli and tensions and pressures that affect a person as he grows up.
- But in many cases the same flexibility that caused the system to develop a problem will work to resolve that problem if we change the conditions, apply the stresses in a different direction.

To understand how true it is that your eyesight alone does not make up all there is to vision, take this situation: You are carrying a trayful of glasses filled to the brim from your kitchen to your guests in the living room. You manage not to spill as you move over the plastic tile floor, but you are worried about having to step up a little when you get onto a layer of thick carpeting. Rather than risk a misstep, you go more slowly and feel with your foot where the edge begins. As your foot makes contact, you have a mental image of where the carpet is, although the tray hides it from your sight. All the while you are looking at the full glasses and your eyesight tells you that the liquid is level. But suddenly you hear a trickling sound and then your thumb feels moist. Although you still cannot see which glass has spilled, your other senses have overruled the information from your eyes. Your mental computer has figured out that the tray could not have been as level as you had thought, and you start to make balancing adjustments.

That's a crude example because it represents a special situation. In actual fact, the principle of head-to-toe vision applies even in the most sedentary conditions. You may think that only your eyes are at work when you sit reading in a chair. But even then, there is a steady input of other information to the mental computer, telling it about your position. If some unsuspected device should tilt your chair to one side by a very little bit, the oddity of reading slightly uphill and of feeling unbalanced would confuse the mind enough to cause you considerable discomfort after a few minutes, perhaps even nausea. That would be the computer's way of trying to end a baffling situation that made it want to light up "TILT."

So vision is not at all a matter of the eyes alone. Most persons are born with a beautiful pair of eyes, perfectly ready for the job they will be asked to do. But as they send their messages to the brain and get billions of instructions back from the brain and try to mesh in with a whole body system that is operating in conditions of civilization that are unnatural to our outdoor bodies, the eyes and all these other parts are forced into many adaptations in order to survive.

The work of the great research scientist on the glandular system, Dr. Hans Selye, was one of the greatest stimuli to this new view of the visual system. Selye showed how all living things, and therefore all parts of our bodies, when subjected to prolonged stress, must either adapt or die. If, for example, we have to live in extreme cold for very long periods and with scanty clothing, we either form a heavier layer of body fat and a circulatory system that supplies more blood to the outer parts of the body or else we die. If we use one set of muscles violently every day, we either build them up or break them down. Can the eyes be a complete exception to this rule? Classical theory of sight said yes, comparing the eye to a box camera that has a lens, an enclosed chamber, and a retina (which is like the film in a camera). All these characteristics, the theory went, are determined by our genes before we are born.

Now, although our knowledge of the eye is full of gaps, we know that the hereditary shape *doesn't* control everything. We know, for instance, that there are many simultaneous tiny movements going on in the eye which have a lot to do with making some persons see far more than others with the same measurements. The eye is always making minute scanning motions—many per second—to go over and over the object it sees and clarify and refine its findings. The retina itself appears to be more than a mere film to receive light. It is so closely linked to the brain that some specialists say it *is* part of the brain, that it forms some on-the-spot conclusions before passing its information on to the brain for processing.

So the visual system *is* subject to the laws of stress and change that govern the rest of the body. It is, in fact, the most flexible part of all. It is undergoing constant pressures as we go through life—most of these merely reinforcing the system in its old ways because most people keep repeating the same habits. But change the environment or the conditions, and in many cases the vision will change. It has sometimes been said that "you are what you eat." It is much more nearly true to say that "you see according to the way you live."

CHAPTER 2

What Eyeglasses Are for— and What They're Not for

Eyeglasses have become a confusing subject in recent years, and you deserve a simple explanation.

Many years ago it used to be taken for granted that anyone who didn't see sharply needed glasses of some kind. The earliest spectacles were to help aging people see better for close work. Then lenses with different shapes were created so that people could see clearly at a distance. And it was Benjamin Franklin who came to the aid of people who have both problems; he combined the upper halves of his distance lenses with the lower halves of his reading glasses—creating the first bifocals.

At the beginning of this century, a doctor named Bates began to explore the idea that the eyes might be improved by means of exercises, eliminating the need for lenses. He inspired many patients to throw away their glasses, and a good many of them seem to have been convinced that they were happier with the change. Bates was on to some vital truths, and he did us all the great favor of turning a spotlight on the old ideas. But like many pioneers, he made some major errors in his thinking. He worked up an unacceptable theory to explain his successes; and he made far too many claims, leaving himself open to sharp attack by his fellow doctors.

Bates' thinking stayed alive, however, and was pursued by a few practitioners. This school of thought—called "sight without glasses"—excited periodic bursts of interest two or three decades ago, especially when some well-known persons testified to their own sudden improvement. The approach was not yet sound or scientifically thought out, but the public enthusiasm for it reflected a dislike for the old attitude that poor vision should be accepted with resignation even in an era when progress was the watchword in other branches of health. People clearly were not happy with the negative approach.

Today the layman may be confused by the fact that optometrists who believe in visual training and deplore the old approach to eyeglasses do very often prescribe lenses for their patients. In fact, we often advise preventive lenses for children in order to spare them a lifetime of wearing stronger and stronger glasses. Let me explain:

Eyeglasses have traditionally been used as a crutch. They were not supposed to cure or prevent a visual problem. They were not even designed to keep a problem from becoming worse. They were simply supposed to relieve the eye mechanism of part of its focusing task. Like any crutch, such lenses encourage a further weakening. Let anyone lean on a crutch for a while and he will need more and more aid as time goes on. There are many denials that this is equally true of eyeglasses, but we all know that people who wear them usually have to get stronger lenses pretty regularly.

I am not completely ruling out this traditional use of a lens that just helps a person to "see better" with glasses on. If a person just doesn't see adequately to get his daily work done, we have to provide a way, even if only temporarily, while trying by other means to bring about improvements. Some patients aren't motivated to try for visual improvement anyway. A pair of glasses or contact lenses that will make them comfortable is all they want. If, after I explain the various alternatives, that proves to be the case, I do prescribe a lens that is really a prosthetic aid—making sure that it is a minimum correction, not at all an *over*correction, as lenses too often are. In other words, the lighter the crutch that a patient learns to lean on, the less pronounced its debilitating effect will be.

But most of the lenses that many of my colleagues and I have been prescribing for nearly twenty years are not a crutch. They are not prosthetic devices. The principle they work on is totally different, sometimes exactly the reverse of a crutch, for they may actually encourage the visual system to go to work.

There are three types of non-prosthetic lenses that we use—*primarily to lessen the stress of close work:*

- Preventive
- Protective
- Developmental

Preventive lenses may be given to the child who has no visual complaints, but who appears—after an examination—to be under the kind of near-point stress that will shortly produce a problem. This is often found between the ages of six and ten. A "counterstress" lens that lessens the strain of reading will usually prevent that trouble from becoming a reality.

Protective lenses can be provided for the person who does have a visual problem—to preserve at least his present abilities, to protect his eyes from worsening. There are many forms of protective lenses, depending on the nature of the problem. Basically, they are lenses which allow the patient to get along within the existing problem—and with no more stress.

Developmental lenses often are much like the preventive ones—of a type that lessens the stress of close work —but they are used by persons who want to enhance their abilities. These patients may not have any "problem," as such. Often they are people who want to develop the visual system in order to accomplish more in some chosen field or avocation. When used in connection with visual training, the developmental lenses multiply and prolong the effects of the exercises performed during this training period.

For training sessions, the special lenses we use can be stronger than what we prescribe for use outside the office. They are similar in principle, but with a stepped-up effect because they are used in brief bursts and under supervised conditions. What we give a person—child or adult —to take home with him is always on the conservative side.

To give you a concrete idea of the difference between the old-fashioned approach and the modern one, take the case of a child who develops myopic tendencies. This nearsightedness can come from many causes. The older view is that the cause is hereditary, but this actually constitutes a rather small minority of cases. More often trouble seems to develop from doing near-point work under stress—such as reading a lot when the subjects to be learned are difficult. I'll take up this particular problem later on in the book. Whatever the cause, most eye doctors still tend to prescribe a pair of "minus" lenses, meaning a lens that is concave—or thinner at its center—and therefore makes distant images seem smaller, more compressed, more intense. This lens, in other words, is doing

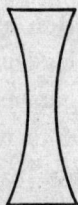

(*Top*) Concave "minus" lens. (*Bottom*) Convex "plus" lens.

some of the focusing that the eye's own lens should be doing. Glasses used in this way never result in completely normal vision.

Assuming that the child's problem is only on *distance* vision, that he sees all right at reading distance, such a lens is especially damaging when used for close-up looking. This happens constantly in school. A child is given this minus lens to help him see the blackboard; but he must also look alternately at the books and papers on his desk. That means his own focusing system is forced to overfocus. The system must adjust further in the direction of myopia in order to overcome the effect of the concave lens. At the very time that study and recitation are causing stresses that make his eyes want to take the easy way out, such lenses encourage him to become a visual cripple.

When we prescribe eyeglasses for preventive or protective purposes, on the other hand, we are pushing the system in just the other direction. If there is the faintest sign of a potential problem, we prescribe a preventive "plus" lens—convex or bulging outward at the center—for close work. Note that this is the opposite of the usual minus correction. We often suggest that the glasses be bifocals. Some families fear that neighbors and other children may scoff at this, but I believe the approach is becoming common enough so that almost everyone will come to accept it as a temporary preventive measure—certainly far less troublesome than braces on teeth. The top portion of the lens is often just "window glass" to allow the child to look up and see the chalkboard without constantly removing his glasses. Only the lower part has the close-up lens.

If the nearsightedness has already advanced to a point where it is hard to see the board or anything more than a few feet away, the bifocal prescription is even more critical. It enables us to give the child a distance lens up top, so that he can look up and see the board without strain, and a close-up lens below that will discourage a myopic reaction when he looks down.

This is just one example of how subtly glasses must be prescribed to avoid harmful effects. What would be a preventive or protective lens for one person might be a damaging crutch for another. It is a matter of first analyzing the patient's inner problem—the adaptation his visual system has had to make in the past—and then prescribing whole new ways of seeing that will turn this tendency along a constructive path.

The question remains in many people's minds, "Can I or my child get rid of glasses entirely at some point? Is 'sight without glasses' ever possible for somebody who has needed them up to now?"

The answer is yes for many cases, but not for all. The kind of preventive glasses I have just been describing, coupled with a period of visual training, often results in the end of eyeglasses for all except close work. My colleagues and I have become quite used to having a young student come in for a checkup after a period of training and telling the child, "Well, your eyes test just fine now. I don't see any reason for you to wear distance glasses any longer." And more than once the answer comes back, "Oh, I knew you would say that this time. I've been seeing much better for the last two weeks."

But we are far from having all the answers, and not everyone who wears glasses can get rid of them and still function at the peak. I like to take the emphasis off of "sight without glasses." If that's the only goal, for purposes of appearance and comfort, most people can wear contact lenses anyway. But the real aim should be *good vision*—the best co-ordinated performance of eyes, mind, and body that today's level of science can provide. Many persons, even with 20/20 vision, perform better when they use mild lenses to lessen the stress of heavy near-point concentration. Many in their middle years can actually slow down the bad effects of middle-aged sight by wearing lenses. Many nearsighted people can be kept from getting worse, but can't yet be cured to the point of throwing away their glasses.

That's why the question is not: Glasses or no glasses? The question is: Glasses for what purpose? When we try to create a new way of seeing for an individual, we must try to ensure that he operates in this new way for most of his waking hours. Exercises alone can occupy only a small fraction of his time; lenses can prolong the good effects. So glasses, which used to be solely a sign of something wrong with the eyes, now become a tool for making things *right*. Their effect on the behavior and the future of the patient behind the lenses is what counts.

CHAPTER 3

What Is Visual Training?

"Visual training contributes to greater achievement, greater safety, happiness and increased self-confidence," in the words of Dr. E. B. Alexander, president of the Optometric Extension Program Foundation.

And another of modern optometry's leaders, Dr. A. M. Skeffington, says: "Visual training allows a person to observe more, see more, remember more, and learn more."

Notice the words . . . greater . . . greater . . . increased . . . more . . . more . . . more.

Visual training is not simply a way to solve a problem. It is a way to surpass, to excel, to achieve, and to enjoy *more*.

The subject is not new. Various limited applications of it have been in existence for a long time. But as the understanding of vision has deepened, the procedures used in training have been elaborated, the criteria for accepting or rejecting a visual-training patient have been sharpened, and the whole standard of judging what constitutes success in such a program has been refined. The positive goal of enhancement has taken over from the former negative approach of merely attacking problems.

The earliest attempts at visual training were directed at the problem of strabismus—crossed eyes. Because it was thought to be a muscle problem and not a defect of the inner eye, it seemed likelier that exercises might correct it, even when other conditions were believed to be beyond help. The techniques developed for this purpose —either as an adjunct to surgery or as a substitute method —were given the name of "orthoptics," meaning "straight eyes."

Just as an example: Let's suppose that a child's left eye tends to drift and to be "lazier" than the right eye in trying to see. One possible orthoptic exercise is to give him a pair of eyeglasses that have a red lens on the left eye and a green one on the right. Then we ask him to look at a slowly rotating disk in front of him, this disk having a geometric design in red and green. He will very likely see all the green portions strongly because his better eye is looking through the green lens; but at first the red objects will tend to fade out, meaning that his weaker eye is not taking part. So we ask him to keep trying to concentrate on the red portions, trying to keep them in sight, and counting the number of times that they fade out. In this way, his left eye is made to put up a fight and we can actually measure the improvement as the number of fadings lessens in succeeding visits.

But visual training consists of far more than orthoptics. Just having the eyes work together and look straight is no guarantee of performance. Visual training is a rounded approach to integrate eyesight, mental development, and control of the nervous and muscular systems. It is not aimed only at eliminating what is wrong, but at developing a more effective and efficient system. The program is designed to build a better "computer." It aims at maximizing "degrees of freedom," to use the optometrist's term, meaning the freedom to engage in the most complex operations with the least stress.

The difference between a retarded child, to take one extreme, and an all-round high achiever lies in the amount of complexity that each one can cope with. Even the very slow child can do some simple operations—perhaps even do them well. If he grows up in that way, it may be said that he can do a routine job, but nothing more. By that we mean that any job involving variables, sudden challenges—whether mental or physical—would be beyond him because his mental switchboard can't handle enough connections at one time to understand and deal with a complex pattern. Most persons are between the two extremes. They can cope with a steady flow of complex problems, but they feel under constant strain. They are always torn between trying to achieve their goals despite this unpleasant pressure or giving up and living a more mediocre life.

The visual system plays a huge part in all this: First, it is the brain's main hope of taking in enough information and experience to stock the mind with "knowledge." Second, it is the guidance system that allows the operations center in our heads to put its knowledge to practical use. Eyesight—movement of hand and eye—movement of the entire body—these are the practical ways that a person turns his thoughts into acts. Trying to do this with an erratic visual system is like a good airline pilot trying to land in the fog with a badly adjusted radar and a set of inaccurate instruments. Would you like to be in that plane?

To pursue that analogy for a moment, if such a plane is brought into the hangar after a series of bumpy landings, its whole guidance and navigational system has to be tuned to work in concert. In just that way, when a child or adult comes into my office with a record of either lower achievement than his heredity and environment should warrant or of having to expend far too much energy in order to achieve, I assume that his visual system may need adjustment. True, his difficulties may all stem from a single flaw; but our nerves and muscles are so flexible that the flaw has almost certainly warped many other parts of the system by now. At any rate, just like running an instrument check on a plane, I have to find out not just what he sees on an eye chart, but how he performs some basic tasks.

It is especially important to know the patient's motivation. A person who just wants to get rid of eyeglasses or who wants to pass an eye exam to enter the Air Force is not likely to be a good candidate. He may get the short-term improvement he is after, but if he is not essentially dissatisfied to live with an inadequate visual system, he is not apt to hold the gains. Someone who wants to *do* specific things well—read, excel at a sport, drive a car, fly an airplane—has an excellent chance. So has the person who has just never given in or adapted to poor vision—one who feels constantly uncomfortable with his nearsightedness, astigmatism, or whatever his symptom may be.

Motivation is one of the key factors, for the optometrist cannot *make* a person improve his vision. He can only give guidance, lay out the course to be followed. Really good vision is *learned,* just as truly fine diction or superb athletic form is learned. Visual training is a process of *learning to see better,* and as in every field, it is always the student who must do the learning. Wanting to learn is the very first requirement.

When someone begins to take visual training, what he starts to learn is a whole series of *visual abilities.* Vision is not like snapping a still picture. It is an ongoing, unending process of coping with movement. The eyes must be controlled to stay on target, they must change focus instantly, their signals must be integrated and interpreted and used as the basis for new eye movements.

So we set up a great many devices to simulate the visual challenges of ordinary life. Some are as simple as rotating disks and a swinging ball suspended from the ceiling; others are sophisticated and complex instruments. All are aimed at heightening the many skills that you unconsciously combine in the process of seeing. Some of those skills are:

The ability to follow a moving target smoothly and accurately with both eyes. This might be a ball in flight, the moving part of a machine, or cars coming toward you as you cross the street. This "pursuit ability" is constantly in use whenever you are out of doors, and often in the home, school, or office, too.

The ability to fix on a series of objects quickly and accurately with both eyes. This is the skill that enables a person to run down and check a list of figures, to see many different numbers on a scoreboard, to get the information from a map or blueprint.

Ability to change focus quickly and without blur. We all have to do this if we drive a car and look from the dashboard dials out to the road ahead. In that case, it can be a life-and-death skill, as it is to the aviator. But it is also an essential in every sport and a basic part of all comfortable living.

Ability to use both eyes together. Although many persons get along without perfect teamwork between the two eyes, it means that a constant conflict is going on inside them. The conflicting information they get from either eye struggles for first place in the mind, and one eye or the other ends up by being suppressed in certain situations. This reduces the total amount of information these persons can take in, lowers their efficiency and sometimes their physical safety. Moreover, it creates a constant drain on their energies.

Ability to see and recognize in a flash. The person with truly good vision recognizes familiar people, objects, and situations in a tiny fraction of a second. Only since World War II has it been realized that such recognition occurs without really "seeing" in the usual sense of getting a full picture of an object. A few prominent contours or highlights give an impression that the mind then interprets from memory.

Ability to integrate body movements with vision. As I have mentioned before, movement is basic to vision. Not only are most of the things we see in motion; the eyes must also be in motion in order to see. And we ourselves are usually in motion while we are seeing. The movement contributes to the way we see, and our vision contributes to the way we move.

So we set up a progression of skills—beginning with simply seeing and following the object visually, then adding a hand movement. Eventually, even more body activity is brought into play, for this is the way vision works in real life—as a guide to complicated, many-faceted movement.

Most of these exercises are done while wearing training glasses—simple convex lenses that help the eye to relax for near vision, but present a slight obstacle for it to hurdle on distance vision.

In my own office I also have a metronome ticking at 120 beats per minute during almost all exercises. Many of the procedures are timed to this—the trainee being told to do one thing for four beats, shift to another for the next four, etc. But even when there is no direct connection, the underlying beat of the metronome helps to build in a feeling of rhythmicality .that is essential to smooth-working vision.

The value and importance of visual training is much better recognized by those who have already had it than by those who need it. Most persons, unless they are actively oppressed by a vision problem, fail to realize how far short of a smooth performance they may fall in most activities. Faulty seeing causes hesitation, discomfort, and endless repetition. This inefficiency is a trickling type of waste, so it is not noticed, but it adds up to a great loss of energy in the course of a day—a great weight of accumulated frustration. Viewed in that light, it is no exaggeration to say that visual training can open the door to a new and exciting life.

For information on optometrists in your area who specialize in the approach discussed in this book, write to:

Chairman, Committee on Orthoptics
and Visual Training
American Optometric Association
7000 Chippewa Street
St. Louis, Missouri 63119

CHAPTER 4

Vision Begins at Home

Habit is what molds us, makes us all what we are. A person's character, for instance, is shaped by the way he behaves most of the time, not by a set of company manners that he puts on now and then. That's exactly how it is with vision: Your basic seeing habits are practiced so constantly that they far outweigh the few hours of special work an optometrist can give you.

This makes it vitally important to be sure your living and working arrangements tend to be good influences. This doesn't apply only to a person or family with overt problems. The principles I am going to outline are even more useful in preventing trouble.

It's like home dental hygiene to provide the day-to-day environment that helps the dentist to keep your mouth healthy, or like having a sound diet in order to make the doctor's treatment more effective. Vision is even more continuous than either of these things. You brush your teeth twice a day, eat three times a day. But you're working your seeing system every waking moment.

Here are some practical arrangements that you and

your family can use to minimize the stress on each member's eyes:

Lighting. Avoid sharp contrasts in light: This is an important rule to keep in mind wherever visual tasks are being performed.

Working with just a desk lamp is very unwise. The whole room should be illuminated. If a desk lamp is used in addition, be sure that the bulb is shaded, so that the eye isn't exposed directly to the light. If the lamp is

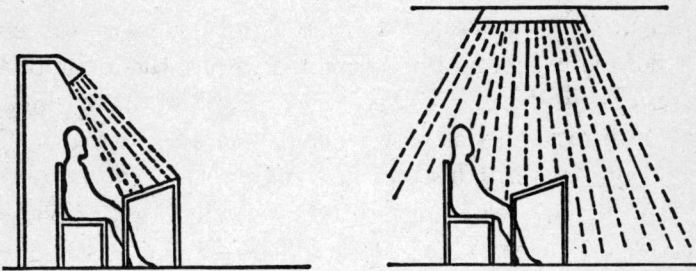

(*Left*) Poor lighting—centralized light. (*Right*) Good lighting —evenly distributed light.

fluorescent, it should contain at least two tubes. And in any case, make certain that it doesn't create a strong glare in the work area. Here is the reason:

The eyes will always tend to center on the location of sharpest contrast—drawing them away from the task demanding attention. The result is steady stress. If contrast is reduced, stress is reduced.

For a similiar reason, you should avoid writing on white paper that rests on a dark mahogany desk. Either use a desk with a light finish, or put a blotting pad of an intermediate shade under the paper in order to reduce the contrast at the edge of the paper.

I will not comment on the amount of light needed, in terms of watts or foot-candles, because research has shown that this is not as important as what are called "the brightness factors." These include the amount of reflecting that is done by all the surfaces in the room—walls, floors, desks, etc. Light-colored walls and ceiling obviously call for less total electric power than a room with dark or heavily draped surfaces. Personal comfort of the people in your family must determine how many lights you need in each room. In most homes, what is needed is not more lighting but a reminder to *use* the lights that are already there. Wherever visual tasks are being done, turn on the lights as soon as any dimness is sensed—and turn on several lights, not just one.

Ideally, the area immediately surrounding the books or papers being looked at should be lit just as brightly as the work itself. There can be some difference without causing trouble, but if the ratio gets anywhere near three to one, the visual system is put under considerable stress. The peripheral environment also plays a part—the farther reaches of the room. Scientifically, a ratio of ten to one is considered the outside tolerable limit; that is, the far corners should have at least one-tenth as much light as the desk or worktable. Since it would be a nuisance to make precise measurements, let's just say that no part of the room should be in deep shadow.

Does all this mean that the modern decorator's idea of having only lamps in the living room should give way to the old-fashioned ceiling fixture? No, several lamps usually provide adequate light for social purposes. Over-all lighting is a must only when there is intense concentration and use of the eyes. Even in that case, lamps are acceptable if they are the type that give indirect light, that is, beam the light up toward the ceiling and let it reflect over the whole room.

TV Watching. This can be a perfectly healthy pastime if it is done properly. In fact, the knowledge and vicarious experiences that can be gained from the better programs are a help to general development. But television should not be allowed to become a "baby sitter." These basic rules are important:

• Other room lights should be turned on—about the same amount of light you would use for general company conversation. This is critically necessary for the same reason that we have just been discussing above. Looking at a TV screen is identical to staring into a low-power light bulb. The contrast must be reduced by having light all around, with the lamps carefully placed to avoid any direct reflection on the screen.

• Sit far enough away so that distortions and electronic flashes are not noticeable, but not so far away that there is any straining to see the details. Watch young children especially on this, for the younger the child the closer to the set he will tend to move.

• Don't become "glued" to the TV. Adults normally move away from the set often enough to break any excessive concentration. But here again, children have to be watched a little more carefully. If you speak to someone who is watching TV and get no response, it's likely that the person is, in fact, too deeply engrossed and should be interrupted.

Furniture, Colors, and Room Arrangements. What I am about to say applies only to rooms in which close work is likely to be performed. The size and color of furniture, the posture that it promotes, is vitally important to your family's vision. But this does not mean that every room in the house must be arranged with special attention to this aspect of health. Far from it—pleasant and inviting rooms are more important than achieving laboratory conditions.

In the areas where a lot of reading, study, sewing, or close-work hobbies will be going on, however, some extra care will pay big dividends. In addition to what I have said about the lighting and the need for light-finish furniture, it is helpful to keep wall colors soft and to avoid sharp contrasts of color. Such contrasts tend to fight for a person's attention, even when he thinks he is concentrating on the task at hand, and so they cause an unsuspected stress—analogous to the fatiguing effect of trying to converse against a background of continuous noise.

Equally important, the furniture used for close work should enable a person to maintain proper posture. By "proper" I do not mean the straight back that is usually associated with that term. The right posture for a near task differs from the posture for a distance-oriented one. The chair must permit feet to be flat on the floor (otherwise phone books or a box should be placed under the feet). The desk or table should be at about waist level when a person is seated; a child working at a surface that is too high for him gets as much distortion as you do when you see a movie from a side seat way down front. A round "O" looks blimp shaped, and all other letters and objects are similarly warped.

•Whenever possible, the work surface should be tilted up to about a 20° angle. When this is done, and the head is bent slightly forward toward the work, the plane of the face will be approximately parallel to the book or paper. Incidentally, the ideal distance from eyes to reading matter can be gauged by making a fist and measuring the distance from the middle knuckle to the elbow—which is about fourteen inches for an adult. Whatever the measurement shows is a good reading distance for that person.

You may be able to make your own tilted work surface or to get a nearby hardware store or handy man to make one for you, by nailing a smooth, flat board onto two supporting boards cut into elongated triangles, like this:

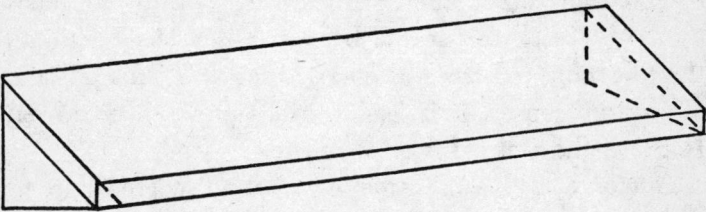

Reading in Bed. I'm sorry to say it, because reading in bed can be very pleasurable, but it *is* usually harmful.

This is especially true when a person is ill, particularly with a high fever. At such times, both reading and TV watching should be avoided. I know that that creates a problem of "what can he do with himself?" But it's less of a problem than being left with a visual condition. I sometimes suggest that the patient take the opportunity to rediscover the value of radio.

Even under perfectly healthy conditions, reading in bed puts all kinds of warps into the visual system. I cannot emphasize too strongly how important posture is to vision; the reason is not very mysterious. To over-simplify, we can say that the brain and the whole nervous system get attuned to working in a certain position and it becomes "normal" for that particular system. If that "normal" state for a certain young person is based on long hours of being curled up in bed, lying on one side, propped on an elbow, the eyes not even level with the print being read, what happens inside the system when this person sits at a school desk or stands to recite or grows up and starts to drive a car? These are all "abnormal" positions for his particular body. Reading in bed or doing any other intensive eye use while ill multiplies the bad effect because the body is absorbed in fighting the infection and has less energy than usual for fighting off odd influences. It is likelier to adapt, to give in even faster to the warped way of seeing.

Out of Doors. Most Americans spend a large part of their lives outside and may wonder what effect bright sunshine has on their vision. The answer is that bright sunshine, as such, is neither good nor bad; but if it creates discomfort, then the eyes need to be protected from it.

Generally speaking, I do not prescribe sunglasses for children unless they are definitely complaining. The reason is that we like to maintain the widest possible range of freedom to adapt to different light conditions—especially in the formative years. So when a parent asks about sunglasses for a child, I always try to find out whether the child himself has ever shown signs of discomfort in bright sun. If not, I advise against sunglasses.

For grownups, whose sophistication makes them more aware of sharp changes in light intensity, I think the proper sunglasses or tinted lenses are an acceptable addition to comfort—but again only for use when the sun actually causes annoyance. Use of sunglasses in moderate light, when there is no real need for them, has nothing to recommend it.

Let me make a careful distinction between bright sunlight and *glare*. While sunlight alone is never harmful, a real glare is another matter. People who do a lot of boating, fishing, or winter sports and who frequently notice glare should be very careful to wear protective glasses—usually Polaroid, since the directional nature of the glass cuts out direct reflection.

I should mention, too, that the quality of sunglasses is important. The ones that do not contain optically-ground lenses can sometimes have irregularities that distort the vision—not usually enough for the wearer to notice, but enough to have a bad long-term effect. Paying a little more—not for the fancy frames, but for the lenses—is usually a very worthwhile expenditure. To be absolutely sure about sunglasses, it's best to get them from your optometrist, even if you don't need a prescription for distance vision in them. If you already have a pair, at least ask him to check the lenses—a simple procedure that requires only a few seconds.

Of course, I have been able to cover only a few of the daily arrangements and activities that make up your life. But you will find that the *principles* behind these suggestions can be applied to many other situations. The lighting rules that are best at home are also best in an office, even though the types of fixtures may be different. The furniture and posture that is best for reading at home is equally good for close work anywhere else. Once you know what is basically good visual hygiene, you can carry the knowledge with you as a common-sense way of protecting and improving your health.

CHAPTER 5

These Exercises Are for Everybody

I'm going to tell you some of the things I ask my visual-training patients to do at home. These are not to cure any one particular problem. They are to tone and improve the visual system. They are good for persons of any age, and most of them are easy enough to be explained even to small children. Whether or not you have a specific visual problem, these exercises will be of benefit to you. Simple as they may seem, they can be very effective by increasing the smooth co-ordination of muscles that affect the eyes.

I'll begin with exercises that can be done alone, then suggest a few games from which the whole family can benefit.

All of the following procedures are done in a relaxed, well-balanced posture. This means standing with your feet slightly separated and weight distributed equally on either side of the body. One way to achieve this posture is to stand with the feet eight or ten inches apart, then go up on your tiptoes and reach stiffly for the ceiling, so hard that you feel the tension in the back of your legs; then drop down flat on your feet.

One general rule for all these exercises is to stop the moment you feel any disturbance—dizziness, nausea, or any such upset. Record how much you were able to do, then go on to the next exercise.

If possible, you should have a "balance board," which your neighborhood hardware store can construct for you if you have no way to make it yourself.

All that is needed are two pieces of wood—a one-foot length of 2″ × 4″, and a piece of heavy plywood ¾″ thick and 12″ × 18″ in size. The flat plywood board rests on the broader surface (the 4″ side) of the two-by-four, so that it balances. Standing on this board is not for the purpose of developing any trick acrobatic skills. It is to enforce the balanced posture that is so important.

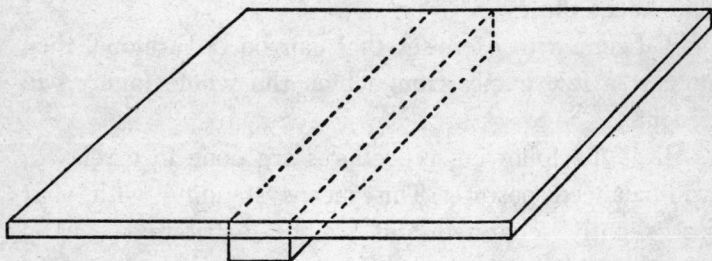

● *Deep Breathing*

Stand in your relaxed posture, preferably on the balance board. Inhale through the nose, raising your head, and pause for three seconds. Then exhale through your mouth, lowering your head, and pause again. If you find that the balance board keeps you from performing properly, get off and continue the procedure standing on the floor. The goal is to do ten deep breaths in this way. But you may be able to do only two or three at first.

• Neck Rotations

This is an old calisthenic used by football players. It is *never* done on a balance board. Standing with your eyes gently closed, rotate your head around your shoulders three times in a clockwise direction, then three times counterclockwise. Open your eyes and look. If there is no dizziness or other upset, repeat this whole procedure three times. That makes a total of nine rotations in each direction as a first goal. When you can do that much easily, lengthen it to four rotations in each direction, then open the eyes and look, then repeat the whole thing a second time and a third—meaning a total of twelve rotations in each direction, punctuated by three openings of the eyes.

Your head movements will probably be rather jerky at first. Make the movement as full and smooth as you can, but do as much of it as possible with the neck, trying not to sway the whole body.

• Alternate Wink

Make a target by drawing a letter in crayon on a plain white 3″ × 5″ card. Place this at eye level and stand back five feet from it, preferably on a balance board.

Then, looking steadily at the target, wink your eyes alternately, up to a total of forty winks. The goal is to keep the target clear throughout the procedure and to keep it stable—that is, it should not appear to jump in position. Whenever it jumps, you are making a slight error in computing the location of the target.

It is very important to introduce a rhythmic pattern into this exercise. If you happen to have a metronome, set it at 120 cycles and use that to set the rhythm.

• Closed-Eye Rotations

Standing, preferably on the balance board, gently close your eyes and imagine that a large disk is rotating in front of you. Picture a big colored dot painted at the edge of it, and follow that dot with your closed eyes. (Another person in the room should be able to see your eyes moving behind the closed eyelids.) Now, at the same time, point your thumb and forefinger and follow the imaginary rotating dot with them, while also rubbing the two fingers against each other. I don't care which arm you use. But I do want you to change direction—so that the imaginary rotation is sometimes clockwise, sometimes the reverse. The time goal here is ultimately to do this entire procedure for one minute in each direction.

• Head Rotations

Stand relaxed, preferably on a balance board, and place the same marked target card you used before at eye level on a wall five feet in front of you. Clasp your hands together at the back of your head. Now, keeping your eyes open and fixed on the target, start rotating the head in a small arc. Gradually, as you are able to keep seeing the target clearly, you will be able to increase the arc of rotation, but this may take a good many sessions. You should eventually do this for one minute in each direction.

• Closed-Eye Fixations

Here we are interested in accurate and rhythmic change of eye position, as would be the case in looking from one object to another. Stand in the proper posture, preferably on the balance board, and with the eyes closed. Then in a definite order shift your eyes as far as you can to right, left, up, and down. It is a help if you have another member of the household call out the positions in a rhythmic sequence. You can change the order from day to day, but keep the pattern the same on any one day. The goal on this is two minutes.

• Four-Corner Fixations

No balance board on this one. Stand five feet from a wall with the eye-level target card in front of you. Put a hand up to cover one eye. Look at the target card for four counts or four beats of the metronome. On those beats you do four specific acts: *Look* at the target; *Point* at the target; *Down* with your hand; *Hold* the fixation. Then shift to one corner of the wall for four beats and the same four actions. Back to the target card again, then look at another corner. And so on, going back to the target before moving to each of the corners. Do it for two minutes, then put the other hand up to close off the other eye and do two minutes more.

Now for a few simple games that can add a little competitive interest to the process of improving your control of eyes, hands, and visual system. Using these basic ideas, you may want to develop more elaborate games of your own.

"What Is It? Where Is It?" This is a game for children, but it can be varied according to the child's age. The child stands with his hands behind him and a familiar object is placed in one hand or the other. By feeling it, he is supposed to identify it. If he is old enough, he is to tell whether it is in his right or left hand. For a child who has begun to learn simple spelling and counting, plastic letters and numbers can be used. As successive ones are placed in his hands, he is asked to identify the sequence or the words they spell.

The "Where Is It?" game simply consists of asking the child to close his eyes and then point to where he thinks certain objects are. This can be played anywhere and any time. For example, at the end of dinner, while various dishes and objects are still on the table, the child can be asked to close his eyes and point toward the sugar bowl, the salt shaker, his father's coffee cup, and so on. This is wonderful practice. Each time he opens his eyes and notes where he is pointing, he will add to his idea of how visual information is gathered and used. But don't tell him that it has anything to do with learning. He'll find out for himself that learning and fun are often the same.

"Pie-Tin Rotations." Standing in the proper posture, preferably on the balance board, hold a large, smooth pie tin with a marble in it. The tin is held with both hands at arm's length and slightly below eye level, so that the movements of the marble can be seen. The trick is to manipulate the pie tin so that the marble rotates continuously and *as slowly as possible.* Do it for one minute in this position, then let someone else try to do it and see who is steadiest. After that, try it while holding the pie tin as far to the right and left sides as you can stretch, but still seeing it with both eyes *without turning your head.*

"Concentration." From a deck, take eight pairs of cards and four single cards. These twenty cards are shuffled and dealt out face down in four rows of five cards each. The goal is to match pairs. As each player takes his turn he selects a card, turns it over exposing it to his opponent, then selects another card to see if it matches. If it does, the pair becomes his property. If not, both cards are turned back face down. Remembering the positions of these cards becomes, of course, the key to succeeding on future turns, so the game is a fine exercise in memory control of visualized objects.

"Missing the Ceiling." In a recreation room, garage, or any room where a bouncing ball can do no damage, try tossing a rubber ball underhand toward the ceiling without quite hitting. The goal is to come as close as possible

without actually touching the ceiling. This requires very delicate control of the arm muscles and depth perception under difficult circumstances, since the ceiling is a blank space that gives few visual clues to its distance. The higher the ceiling the better, of course. You can vary this game by stretching a rope or clothesline about five inches below the ceiling and trying to lob the ball over the line, but just under the ceiling. This enables you to make it a real competition between various members of the family—with each taking a certain number of turns and recording the number of successful tries.

When I get my new trainees together and have an orientation session for them, all in a group, they take to these assigned exercises and games very well. People, whether small or grown-up, usually feel better when they see that others are doing the same general things. Working on this at home, you may wonder, "Can these simple little exercises really make a difference in the way I see?"

The answer is *yes*. They won't cure any major problem all by themselves, but they will invigorate and smooth your visual system in much the same way that simple physical exercises can turn a flabby body into a hard-muscled one. The only reason that such results seem rare is that few persons stick to simple exercises long and hard enough to see their dramatic possibilities. After all, what can be simpler than sit-ups and push-ups? Yet those two exercises alone can produce an iron body if done long enough. There are some Oriental wrestlers who do almost nothing else in the way of gymnastic training, but they do hundreds of sit-ups and push-ups daily.

I don't suggest overdoing it in any such Spartan way. But I want you to realize as you do each of these exercises that their simplicity is deceptive. I have seen their effects on hundreds of patients—seen them mirrored in the form of better school grades, easier reading, disappearance of headaches, superior sports performance, and more graceful bearing.

CHAPTER 6

"What Can I Do for My Child?"

Every parent asks that question—from the moment a child is born until long after he is grown—and the question has turned into, "What should I have done that would have been better?"

On the visual side—which isn't everything, I know, but which does affect almost every other part of living—parents can do a lot to help. This can start—in fact *must* start—in the first weeks of the baby's life.

Two important early pointers are:

- Keep the infant in a room that is usually well lighted.
- Move his crib around to various positions in the room so that he is attracted to light from different sides.

Approaching the baby from alternate sides is important, too, for changing or feeding. It is natural, but wrong, to keep the crib against a wall and to approach the baby always from one direction; in his brand new state, this gives him the impression that he has only one side. As time goes on, talk to him from different parts of the room as you move around, so that he can learn to follow a target. And put him in as many different rooms as possible during daylight periods, so that he sees different patterns of light and many bright objects.

A mobile hanging outside the crib is a useful aid in making the baby alert. Also, the oldest of playthings—a light rattle—gives him a good chance to see, feel, and hear at the same time. Even if he only gives it a shake and drops it almost instantly, don't think it is a waste of time. This is an experience that the new brain begins to store up for future use.

A little later, at four months or so, it's good for the infant to have plastic blocks and other clean, harmless objects that he is free to *put into his mouth*. This is a very important way of gaining experience, since the mouth is the child's most dependable indicant of what a thing is really like. From four months on, you will notice that a child's way of investigating an object is to see it, grasp it, put it to his mouth, then throw it—to get an idea of how far "out there" is. In order to avoid a series of frustrating half-experiences for him, he should not be surrounded with things he is forbidden to put into his mouth—not until he has passed this period of experimentation and can begin to understand the difference between what is allowed and what is not.

It is very important to start playing infant games with the baby at about this same time—four to five months. Patty cake is such a wonderful combination of many right things a young child needs that it should make us all feel suitably humble about the importance of tradition. Although there were serious errors in child development because so much of today's scientific knowledge was simply unknown, that shouldn't tempt us to discard what the past can teach us. Parents can also develop their own games with the baby, or variations of the standard ones—games that involve handing bright objects back and forth, and as much movement as possible. But bear in mind that the movement must be closely related to the baby's own body. He hasn't yet discovered much of the world or how he relates to it. The space he lives in and knows about has to be expanded steadily, but in a coherent way.

At about six months, the infant should be interested in things across the room, objects too far away to be reached with his arms. Now he needs to learn a lot more about size and distances. Just looking won't achieve that. The eyes give us reliable information only about things that we have encountered close up. So we come to one of the most important rules a parent can learn:

Plenty of opportunity to move and eventually to crawl in the widest possible area is vital. Every day—if the room can be made warm enough—a crib sheet should be spread on the floor, and the baby should be allowed to move around with as little restriction as possible. When temperature conditions permit, it is even useful to let the infant move with no clothes on at all. Babies who have been restricted by lack of space or by excessive germ-consciousness on the mother's part are likeliest to have developmental visual problems—crossed eyes, amblyopia, imbalance of the two eyes, etc. All too often, when they leave their crib, it is to move into a playpen or into the type of baby chair that encircles them within a table. Just when they are supposed to learn about the world, they are asked to do it from a jail.

Imagine yourself as having been anesthetized and waking up in a huge coliseum-like structure where all the objects are a block away and unrecognizable, looking like products of another world. If you could keep your sanity long enough to investigate and make some sense of these new surroundings, you would consider it essential to be able to move all around this weird building, to go up to each distant object, touch it, gauge its relative size from close up, move on to other objects. If instead, you were penned in the center, what chance would you have of avoiding a wildly distorted impression?

Well, baby's best chance is to spend a number of hours each day on the floor, moving about as much as his energy dictates. Learning begins with movement, as some of the wisest pioneers in behavioral science have said. This movement must freely integrate all parts of the body— to match sight with feeling.

Imagine then how frustrating the misuse of a baby chair can be. A high chair or the lower kind of chair that has a little table around it can be very useful aids at mealtime. But they must *not* be used as tenders, to "keep the baby out of mischief" for long periods. They restrain his normal motion, and some of them even prevent him from seeing his own feet, cutting his space world in half.

One other infantile object to be strictly avoided is the suction-cup rattle that is attached in front of the baby so that he can touch it, but cannot bring it to his mouth or throw it. (Often it is attached to an enclosed baby chair, to complete the job of restricting this young person.)

When the baby has become big enough to stand and walk about on two feet, it's not too soon to give him the wonderful training that is involved in trying to catch a ball. Since he can't really accomplish that yet, a balloon can be used instead. (But be sure it's a strong one and not too tautly inflated, for a loud bang could cause permanent fear.)

Coming now to the very important subject of toys, there are two kinds of toys for small children: those chosen with the child in mind, and those chosen with parents in mind. When we see that frequent and humorous instance of a child ignoring the toy and playing with the box it came in, we know that it was a parent-type toy. A toy, in order to be fun and instructive for a child, must be a tool that he can manipulate. He is a little scholar, an explorer, a determined investigator. That's his business in life, and that's what he likes doing. We may smile and say condescendingly, "Look how busy that little fellow is," but the joke is on us: because he *is* busy rumpling that paper or opening and closing that box—as deep in thought as any nuclear scientist in a research laboratory.

So toys can be some of the most important influences in a child's life—toys plus a lot of parental attention. Very often modern scientific findings serve only to make us more appreciative of some old-fashioned things that we had never thought much about one way or the other. Now we know that rattles and balls and jackstraws and building blocks are some of the greatest "training aids" a child can have, and that a mother's patient repetition of infantile instructions—"Look for the ball" . . . "Find the pretty picture" . . . "Where's the baby's rattle?"— are often better preparations for life than a lot of the modern parent's half-informed probes into behavioral psychology. Here is why:

A child's great challenge is to learn about the world around him in the way it appears to all the other people he will have to live with. This doesn't sound like much of a problem to us, now that we've got it made, but it is a tremendous job of organization and synthesis to the newcomer. The simplest and most basic objects that we take for granted are actually composed of many facets, and we learn to organize the multiple ideas they represent into one concept. Take a box, for example. Having seen boxes and called them by a single word for so many years, we think a box is obviously a single idea. In fact, it is a collection of separate lines and flat surfaces and angles, of different textures, different colors. In other words, "box" describes a huge family of characteristics that happen to have a common denominator. The child who begins by not even knowing the extent of his own body or how it relates to the world around him has to learn concepts like these by the dozen every day. Then he has to be able to develop the knack of keeping track of scores of spatial relationships at the same time. And this is a trick of vision and memory that is really miraculous. An excellent book called *Success Through Play*, by Don H. Radler and Newell C. Kephart, describes it this way:

"As you sit in a chair reading this book, you must be aware of your location in the chair, the chair's location in the room, the position of the table next to you, and perhaps of the ash tray and the drinks that are there. If you shift your attention from the book to the door when someone enters, you must remain aware of where the book is, so that you can return to your reading without spending ten minutes looking for it. . . . But think for a moment of how the world looks to a very young child who has just begun to know that a chair is to sit in, a Mommy is to get food and love from, and a rattle is to play with. Each time he shifts his attention from any object to any other, he forgets where the other objects are. Thus, you will often see a young child looking for a rattle all over the room while the rattle is in his right hand, or attempting to sit in a chair two feet away and ending up on the floor, amid loud and surprised bawling." Almost every month his problem is complicated by the fact that he keeps growing in size. Things around him seem to shrink in relation to his body.

If for some reason or other a child is a little late in catching on to these spatial relationships and the knack for keeping them all straight in his head, he is soon foundering because new experiences keep crowding in, new attainments are expected of him, and he hasn't yet conquered the old ones. You may wonder what these bits and pieces of development have to do with a child's vision and his achievements in later years. Well, as Radler and Kephart point out, if some of this lag persists when he goes to school, he will have more trouble than normal with such seemingly unrelated subjects as arithmetic and spelling. He will find it harder to understand that $2 + 2 = 4$, because that's a *relationship* among four different objects. He may have trouble remembering that the two letters g and o spell *go* because that's true only if they are arranged in exactly a certain way. A child who doesn't make a firm distinction between left and right might not always put the g and the o in the same place. He might sometimes put one above the other. Or he might be one of the many children who reverse letters as if in a mirror, so that

B is seen as ꓭ
and L is seen as ⅃ .

These problems may seem to be mere trifles to the adult, but they can be a baffling maze to the child.

Don't think for a moment that a young person has to be "slow" to be caught in such a snare. Most of these things that we take for granted, such as spelling, are merely conventions that a segment of society has arbitrarily decided on. The child who doesn't pick them all up at once may be an individualist who goes in less for mimicry than do his peers. He might even be reflecting an above-average talent that leads him to think in original ways. But this is not a good reason for "just letting him alone" if he is obviously suffering from his isolation. We don't have to make him into a conformist—just give him the mental tools that are his birthright. It is highly unlikely, if not impossible, that a superior intellect will be stunted by being given a chance to learn and enjoy at least as much as the average minds around him.

Just being aware of all this from the child's point of view is the parent's main need. Once you know how unobvious these things are to him, you will find many ways of your own to make sure that he catches on. The chief requirement, in most cases, is just to give him a tremendous amount of experience with shapes and movement and distances.

The book I mentioned above—prepared with the co-operation of the Achievement Center for Children and Gesell Institute of Child Development—recommends many types of play that accomplish this end: A game like "Angels in the Snow" can be played on the living room floor—the child, lying flat and stiff and pressing hard against the carpet, swings his arms out in an arc until they meet above his head. He moves his feet apart as far as possible. Then he brings feet together and arms back around to his sides with a slap. The feel of the carpet and the sounds he hears help to fix in his mind the size of his own body and its relationship to space he sees around him. Later on, the growing child can walk a beam, balance on a teetering-board, play pegboard games, follow a swinging ball suspended from the ceiling and eventually try to bunt it with a bat.

Some children go through all these activities so easily that they make them seem unnecessary. For them, the simple games are just a little harmless practice—and a checkup to be sure that everything is really fine. There is no need at all to push them to develop exceptional skill at these motor activities. Adequate and well-rounded performance is enough. Any great emphasis on a single physical skill may, in fact, hamper the total development of the individual—just as many fine athletes, often much more intelligent than they are thought to be, put all their energies into one sport and neglect other interests. But a good many children have problems with one or another of these activities—problems that are usually ended by some patient repetition. If not, if one or all of these things are hard for a child, it is a signal that more understanding attention to his motor development is needed, in order to spare him a long, hard road throughout his school years.

For a fuller set of suggestions about exercises, games, and other activities that will help all the way from the early weeks of infancy to the early school years, I recommend three books that are basic and easy to read:

Mommy and Daddy—You Can Help Me Learn to See is a brief and readable brochure on infant vision care. You can get it free from: Woman's Auxiliary to the American Optometric Association, 7000 Chippewa Street, St. Louis, Missouri 63119.

Success Through Play, by Radler and Kephart, has already been discussed above as a good summary of how play and games can be used to prepare the child for academic achievement. It is published by Harper & Brothers, New York.

How to Develop Your Child's Intelligence, by Dr. G. N. Getman, is a short manual on the practical ways of building a child's vision and intelligence from infancy on into the school years. It describes a great many physical exercises, games, and puzzles that can be arranged at home. You can get it by sending $3.50 to: Research Publications, Box 219, Luverne, Minnesota 56156.

CHAPTER 7

Reading—the Greatest Skill You Can Learn

Think about a COW.

Imagine what a child sees when shown that group of symbols—COW.

• An average four-year-old sees it as three little marks —a crescent, a circle, and a zigzag line.

• A city child who has learned to read visualizes a *picture* of an animal—something found in a book or magazine. With an effort, he can realize that it is big, but his first reaction on seeing the word is to think of a small photograph on a printed page that can be flipped over at will.

• A farm child knows at once that the word "cow" means a very large animal, capable of pushing *him* over if improperly milked, and evoking a memory of certain colors, odors, sounds, and characteristic movements.

As for you, with your education and broader experience, you can encompass all three of these interpretations, of course. Perhaps my mention of a cow sparked even more ideas in your mind. When you read the first sentence in this chapter did you see letters? or words? or did you experience an impression created *by* the words? What color cow did you imagine? How big was she? How far away? Did you think of her in three dimensions, perhaps even envision the other side of the cow? What sort of field or surrounding did you place her in?

This gives you some notion of the diversity of thoughts that even the simplest word can yield to the experienced mind, just as a musically-trained person can turn a few notes into a full orchestration.

The ability to read is not just one more skill. It is *the* skill. Well over 90 per cent of the information we take in comes through the eyes, and much of it is conveyed by written or printed words. Not surprisingly, then, good reading ability is probably the main success factor in today's world. A child's achievement in school and his parents' ability to prosper and fit into the social circles they enjoy are highly dependent on this one skill.

But while everyone can read, few make it into a genuine asset. Many intelligent, normal, otherwise capable persons are shackled by mediocre reading ability. Even simple information is often missed. Voting ballots are marked wrongly, business letters are misunderstood, school tests are failed, traffic signs violated—all because the words of instruction are misread. When it comes to learning new ideas from books or absorbing the sensitive impressions of a fine writer, even fewer persons get the maximum benefits.

Good reading means experiencing the *thoughts* of the writer—not the clarity, size, or shape of the print. It means becoming oblivious to the mechanical aspects, so that the facts or concepts pour freely into the mind.

To help me illustrate my point, please read the fol-

lowing passage of Ernest Hemingway's with a conscious
effort to *see each word clearly*—actually concentrating on
the arrangement of the letters that form each separate
word:

> All good books are alike in that they are truer than
> if they had really happened and after you are fin-
> ished reading one you will feel that all that
> happened to you and afterwards it all belongs to
> you; the good and the bad . . .

Now continue to read, but consciously trying to *see sepa-*
rate syllables:

> . . . the ecstasy, the remorse and sorrow, the peo-
> ple and the places and how the weather was.

And finally try to read this sentence of Aldous Huxley's
with separate attention to *each letter,* seeing its shape
and how it contrasts with the paper:

> There's only one corner of the universe you can
> be certain of improving, and that's your own self.

Even if you had the persistence to finish any one of
those tasks, you didn't really understand the thoughts,
did you? You were *seeing,* probably seeing far more
than you usually do while reading, but you were not gaining information.

Now go back and read the three excerpts for the sake
of their content.

When you saw the shape and arrangement of letters,
you had sight—light energy striking the retina of the
eyes. But only when this phase of the process became

secondary was your mind free to re-create the thoughts of the writers. The more the visual system is trained to work effortlessly at the reading task, the more freedom you have to work at the real object of reading—to translate the symbols before you and then relate those symbols to your own past experiences.

This ability to *symbolize,* to translate thoughts into printed words and then words back into thoughts, is the clearest measure of the superiority that humans have over all other beings. A chimpanzee has a human-type voice box and can make word sounds; he can also be conditioned to respond to a stimulus. But he cannot communicate symbolically or understand experiences that he doesn't share. When we read even the simplest story we are reliving in our own minds things that happened to other persons in places that we may never have seen. This ability to participate vicariously is a supreme human achievement—not to mention the imagination that enables us to embellish and expand the printed words with ideas of our own. For reading is not only the ability to get meaning out of print; it is also the ability to put our meaning *into* the print that we see before us.

The more trained the persons involved are, the more meaning they can get from a few bare symbols. So nuclear scientists, to take the extreme example, can convey years of thought and discovery to each other in a symbolic statement as brief as $E = mc^2$.

All this helps us to realize why freedom to use the visual system at the near point with the least possible stress is so important.

Thinking for now of adults or young people who are near adult years, what should be done to enhance reading ease and ability?

The visual system must always be checked as a beginning step—to be sure that blockages are not standing in the way of improvement. Counterstress lenses may be all that is needed to make reading a much more rewarding experience. In some cases, the person's condition or his interests may make him want the maximum improvement offered by visual training. Such training removes the blocks to the process of visualizing what the printed symbols mean. The reader is fully with the author, rather than still wrestling with the print.

I am often asked about the value of speed-reading courses. Some of these are so commercial that any applicant is accepted, without much regard for his chance of benefiting. This is unfortunate, for where there are visual problems an attempt simply to read faster can be destructive and create even more problems. But some reading enhancement courses are excellent. At their best, they are an extension of visual training, the ultimate use of total vision. I sometimes advise an adult patient, "Now that you have good visual ability, you may want to take a reading course in order to get even more use from your skills."

Georgetown University, of Washington, D.C., which gives one of the finest such courses, has indicated to me that visually trained persons make particularly good students. They get much more out of the course. Visual training alone, according to some of the Georgetown experts, frequently causes reading speed to double and comprehension to increase by 10 per cent. When such a person becomes interested in a reading course, too, the sky is the limit on both speed and comprehension.

CHAPTER 8

Why Some Children Can't Study

Two kinds of reading handicaps that stem from visual causes may blight the lives of otherwise normal, intelligent children:

• Some learn to read, but not how to learn from their reading. They can accurately interpret the print that is in front of them. They can also write and spell correctly. But they don't absorb the thoughts easily enough to be good students.

• Others get stopped at an even earlier point. They don't get the hang of reading at all. They mistake one word for another, spell badly, write miserably.

Children in the first group are sometimes called "near-point underachievers." In most cases, they seemed to do well when they started school, but the stress of close work has overcome their desire to succeed, so that they unconsciously slacken the efforts of their visual system in order to lessen the pressure. It would be wrong to say that they should not do this, that they are lazy. If their systems did not find this safety valve, they might crumple under the strain in some other way. The answer is not to drive them to work harder. Neither are school remedial reading courses apt to help—for it is not reading skill that they lack; it is visual skill. They need visual care—possibly training and almost certainly counterstress lenses to wear while studying. They may also need some tutoring after their ability to study is normal, simply in order to fill in the factual learning that they missed during the period of underachievement.

It is natural for the reader to ask, "What is underachievement?" I prefer to be practical, rather than dogmatic, about defining this. In theory, it means any level of performance that is below that person's potential capability. But that would include almost everybody. There is no known way to measure potential, and no known ceiling to learning capacity. But when a child with successful parents and environmental advantages barely passes or gets only average grades, this is probably underachievement for *him*—especially if it is combined with behavior problems or signs of unhappiness. Without trying to make everyone into a genius, it is surely desirable to cultivate his potential by any reasonable means available to us.

The other kind of perceptual problem that can keep a young person from reading originates in preschool years. It happens to children who were unprepared for the task of learning to read when they started school. There has been a tendency to assume that at age six every child is ready for first grade, and soon thereafter to start recognizing letters and putting them together into words. But development isn't that uniform.

Children mature at different speeds. Girls develop faster than boys. A girl's acuity normally reaches 20/20 shortly before she is six—a boy's not until after six. This is only one indicant of visual ability and by no means decisive, but it is a striking evidence of how wrong it is to expect uniform capabilities at a given age. On top of the natural pace of development built into each child's genes, there are differences caused by environment— the variety and kinds of experiences.

Parents should be aware of how great a help in this direction kindergarten can be. Child-care experts sometimes recommend an extra year of it for a youngster who appears unready for close work, and the parents may feel that this is a reflection on the child's innate quality. But it means only that he needs time to mature some of his mechanical skills.

Kindergarten is where a child can learn about spatial relationships that will help him to cope with the many curious symbols we use to put our language into written or printed form. You will notice, for instance, that the good kindergarten teacher keeps most activities moving from left to right, because that is the conventional direction that our society has adopted for reading and writing. She also makes sure that each child is developing the ability to differentiate form, to distinguish between curved and straight lines. When you see such apparently simple tasks as coloring circles one color and squares another color, bear in mind that this is a step toward identifying letters later on.

Some children who seemed all right in kindergarten begin to fall behind in the first and second grades. A variety of causes can combine to create such problems. "Readiness" is a relative term, for one thing. A child who

seems ready for the first grade may be advanced enough
to do well under one teacher with a flair for explaining
in just the way that comes through to him, but that same
child may fail to grasp a certain basic idea when it is
explained in some other way. And from one or two such
small failures, a whole series of dead ends may result.

Here again, visual training can be one avenue to help.
We can often give the child a new grasp of space and
shapes, of how to use his eyes to figure out the nature of
things. And in addition to training in the office, we
recommend some home exercises that gradually overcome some of the early deficiencies. Just as one example,
a student who is having serious spelling problems after
several years of grammar school may be helped by spelling words *backward* for several minutes of each day. For
bad spelling—which is nearly always combined with poor
reading—means that the child is not really visualizing the
words; he is only taking a stab at them, making approxi-
mations. Being asked to spell "history" both forward and
backward—y-r-o-t-s-i-h—makes the young person really
organize his thoughts about the arrangement of this
word.

The children in this group whose reading problem
stems from an early lack of developmental readiness often do benefit from remedial reading work at the right
time, after their visual skill is normalized. And they will
also need some tutoring to fill in the subject matter that
they missed during the time that they couldn't learn as
other children did.

Of course, prevention is always the best alternative.
Even before the early grades, before kindergarten, the

child is being readied for school every waking moment. I don't mean that two-year-olds should be taught reading at home, as some have suggested. Such premature ventures can even be harmful. And I do not want parents to spend hours of each day on visual training. That would make a distorted life for both parent and child. But just by creating the world a child lives in the parent helps to determine what kind of reader he will be. The language a child hears and the way he plays will be the main factors in deciding this.

Language is the big tie between thoughts and words on paper. "Reading is talking wrote down," as one child expressed it when the great fact suddenly dawned on him. If a child's speech is limited, he is sure to have a difficult time when he comes to reading. Some of the experiences in the "war on poverty" have shown that paucity of language is the main intellectual problem of the very poor. Children who have a very small range of experiences and who hear a limited number of words used are lost when confronted by printed symbols representing words they have never heard and things they have never seen. So a parent can do his child no bigger favor than to expose him to a wide range of ideas and words. Judicious use of television can be a great help in this, although the set should never be used as a baby sitter or allowed to hold the child's attention for too long a time.

Play is the child's main method of developing an understanding of the spatial world around him—the sense of form and direction so essential to reading. A parent should not always be part and parcel of the child's play. But a certain amount of guidance can add to his fun.

Telling one child alone, "Take this ball and go out and play," can leave him with a pretty empty hour. But arranging for a simple ball game he can play with another child or suggesting a solo game that he can play against a wall or with markings on the ground—these small changes can add point and interest to his play. All the activities I have suggested in the chapter "What Can I Do for *My* Child?" will add to a child's understanding of his world and the relationship of objects within it.

We have said that reading is the hardest and most important skill known to man. A child is asked to learn this at the hardest position for man to work at—close-up. He is shown totally different shapes and told that they all stand for the same thing. For example: G, g, *g*, and *G*. He sees these in different sizes, many colors, sometimes clean, sometimes smudged, and he is supposed to sort out in his mind which ones are the same, which are different. After he has learned to read a little, the seven-year-old gets books in various kinds of type, a workbook from another company in different type, mimeographed instruction sheets that look totally different. When he has barely learned to find his way in real life, where objects stand for themselves, he is suddenly shown a mass of symbols that stand for other things—mostly things he has never seen.

It is no wonder that some visual problems or reading problems result. What is truly wonderful is that so many children get through as well as they do. But this remarkable human ability to perform great mental feats doesn't have to be pushed to the limits of tolerance. At a time when the complexity of the world forces children to learn so much more and so much faster than they used to, it is our duty to let them learn under the optimum conditions that we can devise.

The 20/20 Failure

I recently examined a nine-year-old boy whose situation shows why we talk of visual problems in cases where standard eye tests give a normal result.

Fred had seemed to be a bright boy before entering school. He faltered only a little in kindergarten. But when he went into the first grade, he began to have serious problems with simple reading. He showed a pattern of "reversals"—reading *was* for *saw*, and *on* for *no*. In succeeding grades his handwriting and spelling have been very erratic. The teachers have given him "social promotions" each year, but now in the fourth grade the task of reading to learn is all but overwhelming him. He is becoming a loner. He has healthy eyes and 20/20 acuity, but psychological tests have revealed a "perceptual-motor" problem.

The fact is that Fred started the first grade with a handicap. He hadn't developed enough skill at quickly discerning the difference between certain shapes and spatial relationships. The conventional left-to-right direction of most things in our world had not become second nature to him. So some words looked the same to him whether they ran forward or backward. Such small confusions at the very outset make every other piece of learning seem unreal. Fred can never be sure that his understanding of anything is the one that the teacher and most other students have. A program of visual training can teach him to handle the simple visual tasks he should have learned in preschool days. After that, some tutoring to make up for lost information may quickly bring him up to his proper level of ability.

CHAPTER 9

Can Schools Safeguard Vision?

Since teachers and parents are so mutually dependent on each other for co-operation in guarding and developing the child's vision, you will want to know what schools can do along this line. The best way is to tell you some of the things that already *have* been done.

The steps taken in a number of states, counties, and cities indicate a steady trend in the right direction:

Many teachers are becoming aware of visual problems that may exist even in young people whose eye measurements are proclaimed to be "perfect." Superintendents and principals are helping to spread information on this subject, so when teachers find that a student "has just lost interest in his studies," they frequently alert the parents to the need for consulting an optometrist.

More schools are arranging for mandatory visual examinations—which does *not* mean merely reading a chart on a distant wall. This century-old test may indicate, as Dr. Tole Greenstein has said, ". . . whether a child might be a good moose hunter, but not if he can deal with the near-centered task of reading." So the trend is toward a complete analysis of how the two eyes work together, how the system reacts to near-point concentration, how well the person can shift focus between far and near points, and other indicants of practical vision. Such thorough analyses are still far less common in our schools than dental checkups, but a growing number of educators are actively working to remedy this.

A keen interest in "motor development" programs has sprung up in many elementary schools. One of the pioneer examples is Polk County, Florida, where the entire public school system has taken advantage of funds made available by the Winter Haven Lions Club to give many children special rhythmic training and work with geometric forms as preparation for formal learning. Early fears that this might take too much time away from standard subjects have evaporated. It has been proved that the co-ordinated and balanced child learns so rapidly that he more than makes up for the time spent in getting ready. Children who are trained to draw forms, then to combine forms into meaningful pictures, are learning to read, write, and spell with far less problems than any unprepared group. The results have spurred a wave of enthusiasm among many other school systems.

Improved lighting, seating, and other practical arrangements are being more carefully considered when old schoolrooms are remodeled and new ones are designed. The old spectacle of school children with their heads cocked to one side, shoulders twisted, paper skewed around to write at an unnatural angle, is beginning to fade.

Some schools have installed light-diffusers at the windows to make outside light fall evenly from above on all work surfaces, casting no shadows. Many are using soft wall colors, light furniture finishes, and yellow-green chalkboards to lessen sharp contrasts that are harmful to vision and to concentration. Chairs and desks of the proper type eliminate uneven pressures on the spinal disks and intestinal tract that X-ray photographs have shown to be present when school furniture causes improper posture.

Much of this forward movement began with a sweeping project carried out some years ago by the Texas State Department of Health. Dr. Darell Boyd Harmon directed studies of 160,000 elementary-school children and over 4000 classrooms in order to learn how the school environment affected their learning and their well-being. From this, he showed conclusively that light affects posture and posture changes vision. A child at work unconsciously shifts his head and body to fight glare or shadows, and this can eventually warp his skeletal structure and undermine his health, as well as affecting his visual and mental behavior.

Educators who want to review Dr. Harmon's conclusions and specific recommendations for consideration in their future planning can get the information by writing to the Department of Health, Texas State Government, Austin, Texas.

Parents may also find this helpful reading to round out the suggestions for good home-study conditions that I summarized in the chapter titled, "Vision Begins at Home."

The effectiveness of the above seemingly minor changes in school conditions is dramatically shown by

The "square test" in the diagram below shows how a child sitting with his head on one side drew what he thought were a series of squares. This is not just childish inaccuracy. In test after test, researchers found that these boxes look nearly square if seen through a lens and from the unnatural angle adopted by the particular child who made each drawing.

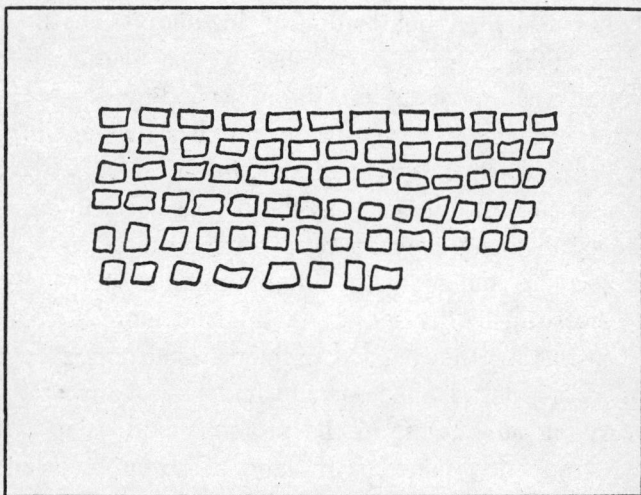

controlled comparisons made during the Texas research. All 396 children enrolled at the Becker School, in Austin, were given thorough pediatric exams, visual tests, and achievement tests just prior to a series of classroom changes aimed at creating an ideal study environment.

That November 53.3 per cent of the children had visual difficulties significantly affecting their schoolwork. Just six months later, in May, all the same tests were given. Only 18.6 per cent of the children still had visual problems—a drop of 65 per cent! Other medical findings also showed sharp improvement, including a big decline in chronic fatigue and ear, nose, and throat infections. The educational achievement tests were equally striking: Without any of these seating and lighting changes, the "educational age" of students at a comparable nearby school rose by 6.8 months during this period. The Becker School children grew an average of 10.2 months during the half year spent under optimum conditions!

So the chance for improvement is heartening; but the over-all problem keeps increasing in one major way: As the pressure for admission at the college level intensifies, schools all along the line raise their requirements. This means more and more reading, cramming, studying under pressure—harder subject matter and more of it.

Considering the massive problems confronting educators in our day, I am happy to find how many of them are taking an interest in the protection of vision. They have frequently joined with men of many other disciplines—with physicians, psychologists, vision specialists, even architects and engineers—to study ways of lessening stress. Such efforts should be multiplied. Most of us who work with vision would wish to see the total hours of study, homework, and required reading carefully regulated at each school level after consultation with an advisory body of vision specialists. For the oldest of educational principles is involved—dating back to Juvenal in the second century A.D. and restated by John Locke in the seventeenth century: "A sound mind in a sound body is a short but full description of a happy state in this world."

CHAPTER 10

The Special Cautions

In your child's life and your own, three kinds of pressures can put the visual system in special jeopardy. Knowing the nature of these hazards and when they are likeliest to appear can help you to minimize their effects:

Preschool Developmental Dangers. From the age of a few months until five years observe the child to be sure the eyes are straight; watch for signs that he might not be seeing well with both eyes, such as tilting the head to one side when trying to see; and take note of how well his co-ordination and balance develop.

Stress of Class Work. Be alert for the first signs of myopia (nearsightedness) in the second grade. In the fourth grade, visual problems frequently take the form of a sudden drop in achievement. Nearsighted symptoms or an aversion to reading and study again become especially common at age thirteen to fifteen. And the last serious threat of myopia comes at age seventeen to twenty.

Stress of Mid-Thirties. It is actually from age thirty-five to forty-five that your own vision needs watching most closely for the symptoms of presbyopia. If the optometrist is permitted to prescribe for this problem even be-

fore it can be called "middle-aged sight," he can minimize future trouble in reading or seeing small objects
close up.

Of course, the ages mentioned above can vary a little.
It is entirely possible for the pressures that hit most children at certain times in life to be delayed for a small
number of others. And a severe illness is a factor that
can usher in a danger period at any time. But there are
sound reasons why the years I have mentioned are the
ones when most persons should have even a little more
attention than usual for their eyes.

The preschool child is constantly vulnerable to the
stress of development, and some of the resulting problems will be discussed in the chapters still to come. When
a child younger than three or four years shows an adverse symptom, we are naturally limited in the kinds of
help we can give. But any sign of trouble should be re-
ported anyway, because the optometrist may quickly
identify the environmental factor that is to blame and
suggest a change that will end the problem at once. Very
early developmental ills can sometimes be nipped within
weeks. Needless to say, any obvious diseased condition—
wherein a child appears not to see at all from one eye or
has some deformity—will also require the attention of the
pediatrician and ophthalmologist.

The next four checkpoints are times of special stress
that is connected with study or other close work. I emphasize again that any year can bring a problem and
that internal stresses can be a contributing factor. But
the optometrist sees too many clusters of cases at certain
ages to have any doubt that they are at least linked to

the stress of unnatural near-point concentration. Most of our school curricula are overloading the visual systems of children, requiring an amount of reading and an intensity of concentration that they are not prepared for. A state-wide study of 160,000 children in the Texas schools some years ago showed that 20 per cent had vision problems by the time they finished the first grade and 40 per cent had them by the age of nine. Less than 2½ per cent of infants start life with defective eyes, so it is clear that the process of just learning to see distorts the vision of more and more young persons as they use their eyes.

It is no accident that the *second grade,* which most youngsters go through at about *age seven,* produces a sudden eruption of myopic tendencies, for this is the first level at which near-point work is a cause of stress to many children. This is the earliest age of concentration, of intensity, of staying with a task, as Dr. Arnold Gesell pointed out.

It is equally apparent why *age nine and the fourth grade* sees another outbreak of problems, usually in the form of underachievement. During the first three grades children have been *learning to read*—which is hard enough in itself. Now, in grade four, with their reading ability still rudimentary, they must start *reading to learn.* This means that a still-unmastered skill must be constantly used for the purpose of attacking other new and mysterious areas of learning. It is as if you had just begun learning French and were suddenly obliged to study nuclear physics in the new language.

In the *early teen years* there are problems of physical

changes connected with puberty. This, almost like an illness, drains off some of the body's energy, so that any outside stress can cause inordinate damage. At just such a time, most youngsters move to junior high school. This involves less supervision by teachers and more personal responsibility on the student's part to keep up, most of which takes the form of heavy reading. Those who are not able to sail through such a period without a big change in their visual systems usually take one of two forks in the road: Either they "adapt" to the new stress by becoming nearsighted—that is, they qualify themselves for the activity that dominates their life at this time; or they shun reading and slip in their studies.

Many a bright student suddenly "falls apart" at teen-age level. The reason is not always visual, of course. There are physical and social problems that can be the root cause. But inability to concentrate on studies, and the consequent sense of failure in school, is a very frequent key. As often as not, the visual acuity is rated at 20/20, so that the parents are told, "There can't be anything wrong with the eyes." I see innumerable such cases, of students with subtle problems that have eluded earlier diagnosis. They get momentary blurring, periodic doubling, headaches, or other disruptive symptoms whenever they try to study for long, yet they have been told repeatedly that there is nothing wrong.

Among the many such cases I have seen in the past few months alone is a girl I'll call Kathy, aged fourteen, who is currently in the tenth grade. As a young child she had trouble with reading, and she later was given remedial reading in the seventh and eighth grades. Her eye exams always resulted in a verdict of "20/20." But although she could force herself to see when she had to, she felt that her vision was often somewhat blurry.

Kathy's grades have fluctuated—tending to be better in minor subjects than in the basic ones. In the few months before coming to me she had tried to improve on this showing and had been reading a great deal more than before. But she found it very tiring, and she was frustrated by the feeling that her record didn't really indicate how hard she worked.

My examination showed that Kathy did, indeed, have healthy, 20/20 eyes. But she had not learned to use her visual equipment properly for concentrated study. Just a few months of training in the right direction was all she needed to fit her for the big job of being a high school student in today's fast-paced America.

The problems of the *seventeen-to-twenty age group* are linked to demands that a sudden change of situation brings about in this period. This is the time when nearly everyone either goes to work or goes to college.

In the early college years the reading load takes one more upward surge—five times as much reading as in high school!—again accompanied by a new sense of challenge and pressure, both academic and social. A good many existing visual problems suddenly become worse, or unsuspected problems finally become major. Students who, without realizing it, have done well through high school mainly as "auditory learners" (listening more than they read) sometimes go to pieces as freshmen when learning from books becomes mandatory.

In most cases it is not reading alone that does the damage. It is *stress*, the drain on bodily energies in several directions at once. It is much like the fact that an attack of pneumonia, which a healthy person can fight off, may overcome and kill someone who was in a weakened state to begin with. A visual apparatus that could cope with a certain amount of light reading during vacation months may collapse under the same amount of reading that is accompanied by mental difficulty and competitive pressure.

But what of the young people who don't go on to college? Many of them can be hit by equally destructive stresses. Even more than the college group, perhaps, they are on their mettle, facing the new challenge of a job. And that job involves very close work a surprisingly large part of the time. Not only the girl who gets a filing job or the eight-hour-a-day clerk-typist falls into this category. It applies to the majority of today's blue collar jobs. The carpenter, the painter, the appliance repair man—all spend long hours concentrating hard on close-up targets.

All the causes and effects of stress that I have mentioned are well substantiated and documented. Not only do our records of elementary school children show these peaks of visual trouble to coincide with new challenges; an even more dramatic example has been repeating itself at the U. S. Naval Academy year after year and has been dubbed "The Annapolis Syndrome." In one class after another, a very high percentage of members (all of them, naturally, young men who entered with good acuity) has been found to be suffering from myopia by graduation time. In one class, more than half of the men became nearsighted! Two lengthy reports on this problem have been published in the *Journal of Ophthalmology,* and the statistics are on file in the Navy Department.

After the seventeen-to-twenty danger period there is a span of about fifteen years when persons are less likely to develop new symptoms. It *can* happen, of course, especially if new demands on the system bring added stress. So normal checkups and precautions are in order. But statistically these years are relatively free from new problems.

Finally, the *pre-middle-age danger zone* is mentioned because nipping presbyopia before it becomes severe can save you from being one of those persons who—while still looking and feeling youthful—has to hold a letter or a menu at arm's length in order to read it, and who then goes on to being handicapped in both near and far vision.

Such a condition may sometimes be aggravated by stresses that are similar to those experienced by the eighteen-year-old—the strain of a new situation. For instance, Morton G., a patient who came to me for the first time in his middle thirties, was suffering from an unusually rapid and acute onset of this "middle-aged sight." I learned that he had been a salesman for all his working career, often out of doors, sometimes on the road. Then at age thirty-five his successful record earned him a promotion to sales manager. Suddenly, at the moment of feeling pressured by the desire to succeed and by all the unfamiliar burdens of executive life, he also found himself at a desk most of the day. A slight difficulty in close-up vision became enlarged into a severe handicap.

As his reading and his pressures increased, the vision problem became more of an annoyance, added to his stress, and worsened rapidly.

Presbyopia is not *caused* by such circumstances, but it is frequently magnified in this way. In Mr. G's case, I was able to arrest the visual decline by giving him glasses that relieved the close-work stress, plus simple training exercises to do at home. But even more of his normal range of vision could have been preserved if he had come just a few months earlier.

During all these special years when the stress of close work threatens most, the best preventive is a complete eye and vision examination at regular intervals. Whenever trouble is diagnosed promptly and lenses or training used to full effect, years of frustration and failure can be turned into successful ones.

CHAPTER 11

The Two Types of Visual Problems

Some of the problems that I am going to summarize for you in the next few chapters are not at all hard to spot —in fact, some are impossible to overlook. But others can go undetected for quite a long time or can appear to be some other kind of trouble.

Since disease and pathological defects of the eyes are relatively rare, most vision problems are not a *direct* threat to health. And it is even rarer for a malfunction of otherwise healthy eyes to cause blindness. Yet such problems, if they are not quickly detected and remedied, can undermine the development or effectiveness of the whole being in a way that is subtle, but *total.*

There are two broad kinds of visual problems:

• Developmental problems occur when a child is deprived, restrained, or restricted during his early months and years. Deprivation, meaning insufficient opportunity to get instructive experiences of all kinds, prevents the visual system from developing adequate skills. Undue physical restraint or restriction causes the start of odd seeing habits in order to cope with the unnatural environment; and these habits warp the malleable young system.

• Stress-induced problems occur later and can be triggered by causes either inside or outside the body. Stress, of course, is a regular part of living. The body, and especially the glandular system, is made to respond appropriately to *transient* stress—to the many calls for a temporary output of energy. But there is no such provision for constant stress. It is steady stress that often causes visual problems.

These stress-induced troubles may result from a serious illness or from the strain of changes within the body during puberty or the middle years. The visual system is not the only one affected during such a period, but because it is such a sensitive one and is usually being worked hard at the very time that body energy is lowered, vision often suffers the most marked effect.

But even without such internal strains, the pressure of near-point work alone is often enough to distort the visual system. The reason is that man's body is essentially made for distance vision. Probably because we are not so many generations removed from the time when our ancestors lived outdoor lives, looking into the distance promotes a relaxation within the body, while close-up concentration causes a real physical strain. Since it cannot live with constant stress, the system adapts itself to near-point work. Sometimes the result of this is what we call myopia: In order to ease the effort of focusing for close-up reading, the system simply gets itself into a chronic "close-up" condition. But obviously a person whose eyes are set and focused for fourteen inches will see a blur when he looks into the distance. This nearsightedness is only one of the symptoms that may show up after a constant stress has affected the individual.

Going back to the first kind of problems—the developmental ones—we find that a lack of adequate and balanced access to information during the formative years can cause even more distress. Here's why:

Suppose a human body, intended by nature to have many sensory inlets for information, pinches off some of the in-and-out traffic through the eyes. The pattern of growth inside this body has to become distorted just like the urban development within a town that is cut off from the highway. Other senses may tend to get built up, mental processes will change to work with the information that is available, actual chemical and tissue changes will take place in the nerve channels—some will tend to wither while others enlarge. The adaptation to this unnatural situation may be a fortunate thing, even a marvel of nature, for without it the body would suffer even more; but the result will rarely be as good as what that body might achieve when working with all its senses.

That's why it is so important to open the child's mind to every opportunity for experience and intelligence that his visual system can provide—and so important to keep the information inlets similarly open and free in ourselves at every age.

I have explained before that I like to think of vision care in positive terms. Although the decision as to what level of care is desired must always be the patient's, it is my duty to let him know that prevention and protection are available if desired, rather than waiting to cope with problems after they have hit. But problems *do* exist, and it is important to discuss the ones that are seen most often—what causes them, how to recognize them, and what to expect in the way of treatment if you consult an optometrist for one of these conditions.

The chapters that follow will give a brief look at each of the commonest symptoms. Bear in mind that all of these are merely the end results of some unseen problem—the outer symbols of whatever is wrong within. We should not think of them as we do of a disease, where we may ask, "What can be done for pneumonia? or tuberculosis? or malaria?" Each of these eye conditions is the body's *adaptation* to a deep inner problem. It is a kind of shield or buffer or device for getting around a problem that is far inside the neuromuscular system. To try to strip it away by some superficial approach—such as surgery or lenses given without a real concern for the root cause—is to deprive the system of a prop without giving a substitute. It can have terribly destructive effects.

CHAPTER 12

When an Eye Turns Inward

Although many visual problems are worse in their effect on the information-gathering system, few cause as much concern as eyes that are out of alignment, because this is the only common ocular upset that is visible and a major drawback to the person's appearance. Probably for this reason, attempts to treat this ailment go back thousands of years.

Convergent strabismus, as the inward turning is called, makes up less than 5 per cent of all visual problems, but it teaches us a lot about the whole subject of vision because it shows so clearly that the person has *learned* to see in a special way in order to meet his conditions. And this makes it vitally important to avoid any approach that tries to wrest from the patient an arrangement he has worked out within himself..

Only very rarely does an inward turning result from pathological causes—from a paralyzed muscle or damage left by a serious disease. The overwhelming majority of cases involve perfectly normal and healthy eyes.

The old explanation is that strabismus usually results from a muscle problem. Those who believe this say that of the six major muscles moving the eyeball, some are stronger than others, so that an imbalance results from the differing pull. This leads to the conclusion that a great many cases require surgery to reattach the muscle tendon at some other point on the eyeball, thereby mechanically "straightening" it.

Many of my colleagues and I favor a totally different approach. We believe strabismus is a functional problem that should be treated on a functional basis. Even aside from the danger always present when a child is anesthetized, we believe that surgery is inappropriate in all but a few exceptional cases, and then only as an aid to the real treatment. That treatment should rely mainly on lenses and visual retraining. For we are convinced that most convergent strabismus is a problem that is manufactured in the process of early development.

There are literally scores of reasons why most crosseyes cannot be ascribed to birth defects or muscle imbalances. I'll touch on only a few.

It is a fact of physiology, for one thing, that a real genetic defect in the body is nearly always accompanied by other defects. It does not seem reasonable that a wellformed person with no other anomalies would have one bad eye muscle. It is not the way nature works. Moreover, the average eye muscle is at least fifty to one hundred times as strong as necessary for the job it has to do. Even a half-strength muscle would be so greatly overendowed for its task that the heavier musculature in the other eye would have little bearing. Furthermore, a crosseyed person can move either eye perfectly well as long as the other is covered; the allegedly weak or strong muscle has no visible effect as long as the two eyes are not trying to work together. And finally, remember that between the two eyes is *bone*. There is no muscular link whatever. The straightness of the eyes is determined solely by the central controls within the brain. The muscles only respond to orders they get from "top management." So to attack the eye mechanically and ignore the brain's role is like doing a wheel alignment on a car because its *driver* keeps veering off the road.

What, then, *is* the cause of inward-turning eyes?

In the vast majority of cases, the symptom is caused by interference with normal access to information and experiences at the very time that the use of the two eyes is being learned. A combination of early environment and habit results in undesirable ways of using the eyes.

You will sometimes hear a parent say, "My baby was born cross-eyed." This is not really so—unless we want to say that all babies are born that way—because there is no significant control of the eye muscles at first. Ocular control begins emerging at four to eight weeks after birth and is not fully established until about sixteen weeks. In the beginning, the orbit of the eye is so small that the iris just about fills it anyway, so it is very hard to tell about eye alignment. And the fact that there is only a fold of skin where the bridge of the nose will be later on can sometimes make even the pediatrician unsure whether the eyes are straight.

After those first three and a half or four months, as the child's increasing control over all his muscles extends to his eyes, the orbit of the eye has become big enough to permit an idea of how the two pupils are aligned. If the parents then finally notice a defect, they naturally believe the baby was born that way.

There are really four specific points in the baby's life when he is likeliest to develop cross-eyes, each apparently resulting from a different phase in the process of learning to control himself and adapt to the world around him. These commonest times are: at about sixteen weeks; at nine months; at eighteen months; and finally at three years of age.

Each of these chronological groups shows a distinctly different pattern of cross-eyes—further demonstrating that the condition relates to the task of getting along in certain activities, rather than to inherited traits.

As examples, I'll mention the symptoms we usually find in the sixteen-week cases and the different traits shown by children whose strabismus develops at age three:

The baby whose eyes are crossed when he is only four months old generally proves, later on, to have good sight in the straight eye while the turning eye is underdeveloped. Very different sets of environmental conditions could account for this, of course. Simply lying on one side in a crib for too much of those first sixteen weeks could be the cause. With one eye buried in the mattress, the other ranges out to explore the room beyond. If this condition applies just when the infant acquires the knack of imposing his will on the eye muscles, he may learn an odd kind of control that freezes this peculiar imbalance into a permanent behavior.

The child whose eye turns at age three often has considerable farsightedness in both eyes. These three-year-old children frequently prove to have great intellectual ability. In fact, cross-eyed children in general are rarely academic problems. Probably the mental keenness that enables them to overcome an environmental handicap by inventing an individual method of seeing also serves them well when they face other challenges. Such children also learn to ride a bike, walk a narrow board, and so on. They adjust their whole motor system to their own pressing needs.

I cannot stress too many times that the crossing of the eyes is, to most of these children, an adaptation they make *instead* of allowing something else to happen. Let's suppose, for example, that the conditions in which the body is developing make it impossible at some point for this child to see the world properly and get the information he needs by normal vision. Many a child, in that situation, just gives up and doesn't get the information at all. Rather than straining any part of his equipment, he just becomes a slow student. Or, frustrated by the confusion he feels, he becomes a behavior problem. But the child who actually forces his eyes into an unnatural position in order to get at the facts is showing a creativeness and an inner gumption that deserves great respect. It also deserves the most gentle and understanding help.

The cross-eyed children who *do* get into co-ordination problems or school problems—and this is most significant —are frequently the ones who have had only surgery for their eyes. Why? Their hard-won adaptation has been torn away, with nothing to replace it. If a child learns to see the world more or less as it is while his eyes are crossed, what can we expect if the eyes are suddenly pulled straight? He will see double, or one eye will just not function. In such cases, the eyes will probably drift out of line again eventually, so that both cosmetically and visually the result will be a failure unless a long re-education of the visual system can overcome the damage.

How can we best avoid all this to begin with?

The key rule is to avoid the interference that causes the eyes to cross—the *deprivation, restriction,* or *restraint* that blocks normal development. Many examples of how to do this are given in the chapter called "What Can I Do for *My* Child?" Some of them may seem too elementary to accomplish such a great goal. But take my word for it that they can make a spectacular difference in the kind of person that will emerge from the tiny bundle of latent intelligence who comes home from the hospital.

Using my examples merely as a guide to the basic principles, you can set up living and growing conditions that give the broadest chance for experiences, indoors and outdoors—all within the common-sense limits of keeping the baby safe from major harm. It will force you to do a lot of footwork and pursuit, to pick up scattered objects, to retrieve balls and rattles. But it's not quite such a boring task, is it, if you are conscious of what's happening inside that lively mind?

What can we do when the eyes are already crossed?

When the problem is brought to the optometrist's attention during the early months of life, the treatment is developmental, not ocular. We point out the need for maximum freedom from restraints. We suggest ways to emphasize the co-ordination of *both* sides of the body, for it is this use of two arms and two legs together that encourages proper use of two *eyes* together. Our suggestions include simple crawling games, pull-ups on the bed with the parent holding the child's hands and letting him pull himself up and let himself down. Also jumping on the bed while holding the parent's hands—to simulate jumping on a trampoline—is marvelous co-ordinative exercise.

When there has not been much time lost and there is little sidetracking of the system to overcome, the cure is often very quick—a matter of weeks or months, at most.

Let me tell you about Ellen, now sixteen years old, to give you an idea of how the treatment of strabismus might go when it is *not* caught at once. Ellen's parents noticed when she was less than two that one eye sometimes "drifted" in toward her nose. She was taken to an examiner who could find no evidence that the eye was turning because the problem was a periodic one and the eye stayed straight in the doctor's office. Some months later the parents were still worried and consulted another specialist—an eye surgeon. He did see the eye turning this time, and he recommended surgery.

Ellen's parents decided to get one more opinion and took the child to an optometrist who felt that the misalignment of the eye was a symptom of a developmental problem. He believed that age three was not a good time to start an all-out training program, since the child was not advanced enough to understand many instructions, and the optometrist feared that any unsuccessful attempt at training might lessen the will to try later on. So he recommended mainly home activities for a time. He prescribed the use of an eye patch—first worn on one eye, then on the other—to keep the two eyes from working together improperly. Later, this was changed to a pair of glasses with part of each lens blocked off—the part nearer the nose—so that the eyes were encouraged to look straight ahead and not toward each other. And he suggested the type of toys, games, and exercises to be done at home that would broaden Ellen's chance of seeing the world in a normal way.

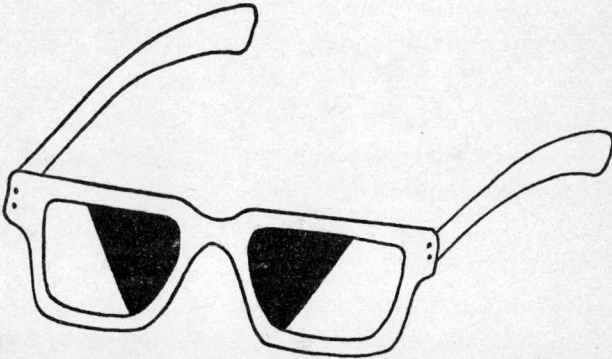

Special lenses with inside halves blacked out, commonly used in visual training of cross-eyes.

Ellen was examined twice a year until she was six, when her family moved to Washington and she was first brought to me. At that point, it seemed time to start a program of intensive visual training in the office. Now she was ready to work intelligently at the various instruments and devices in my office—all designed to give her co-ordination of the eyes and good two-eyed vision. And Ellen was able to learn the *feel* of straight eyes. In order to get this feel, a child must first be taught to cross the eyes on purpose. Most of us can do this by looking inward toward the nose, but a cross-eyed child usually cannot do it. So we have to teach this as a trick—like wiggling the ears or twitching the nose—by moving an object in very close until the sensation of crossing the eyes is linked to a voluntary action and is *felt*. Gradually, Ellen learned to feel if her eyes were straight. From that point on, it was a matter of repeated exercise to hold the eyes straight for as long as possible.

By the age of seven, Ellen very rarely showed any sign of a turning eye, and her vision with both eyes was good. She was given glasses in bifocal form to be used for close work, so that the stress of studying would not cause any new problems to occur. Now, nine years later, she has only routine checkups, wears lenses just for study, and has perfectly straight eyes.

The length of time needed for each case varies widely, of course. Those that are not caught at once and at a very early age often require attention over a long period— three to five years—but it is not continuous treatment. It's usually a matter of periodic training and work at home in between, combined with the use of lenses.

Is there any room for surgery in all this? Yes. There are persons who can straighten their eyes part of the way, but can't quite hold them straight without tremendous effort. This results from the long period of holding the eyes improperly, which gradually does cause one muscle to thicken and bunch up. This is the same reaction you might get from holding one arm up in the air constantly. At first, it would tire. But gradually, it would have to develop a peculiarly heavy muscle to relieve the stress.

When this happens to an eye muscle—as a *result* of cross-eyes, not a cause—I often ask that an ophthalmic surgeon be called in to reposition the tendon and give the eye more freedom to respond to the visual training. We call this "limited surgery," for the understanding surgeon does not try to force the eye into position. He gives it freedom to follow the commands of the brain.

CHAPTER 13

When an Eye Turns Outward

When an eye tends to drift outward, the person is usually taking another avenue toward finding a livable adaptation to the kinds of stresses we have been talking about.

I have often observed a young person in the early stages of reaction to stress seeming to "try out" different ways of adjusting himself to the problem. I have seen a child going temporarily into a phase where one eye turns outward, then finding this to be unsatisfactory, shifting gears and moving into nearsightedness instead. This is often the case when the person's IQ or motivation is so strong that he cannot accept the reduced efficiency that comes with an outward turning. But there are times when these factors are not compelling enough and the person does develop the outward turn that is called *divergent strabismus*.

The strong inner needs that push the eyes in these various directions are strikingly demonstrated by recalling an old approach used in treating this divergence. It was once the accepted practice to prescribe minus lenses —the kind of concave lenses normally used to compensate for nearsightedness. These tend to make things seem smaller, but nearer than reality, so they encourage the eyes to draw *inward*. They often made the person's eye appear straight. But before long the patient was adapting to the artificial situation; either he became nearsighted, or the eye drifted outward again—or both undesirable things happened. For either of these symptoms, the standard treatment was to add stronger minus lenses, and so the cycle became more and more vicious —showing that the person's own way of looking at the world was not being aided at all, but was merely being distorted further by the unfortunate "correction."

This divergence problem, which is less common than the other adaptations we are taking up, by the way, usually occurs in the early school years, in the first and second grades. Most such cases are intermittent, rather than constant, and the student experiences double vision whenever the eye drifts outward. If the symptom becomes more or less constant, there usually is no double vision; the person either adapts himself to seeing a wider panorama or he suppresses the central vision of one eye —using it to see only peripherally. (This enables him to see around a wider arc than most of us, so that some whose eyes are finally straightened complain that they feel as if their vision had been cut off.)

It should be mentioned in passing that there are other variations of these problems in which one eye appears higher or lower than its mate. These need not be discussed separately because they are simply aspects of the same basic situation—a person's attempt to adapt to an inner problem. The optometrist will have to make adjustments in the details of how he treats each case, but the fundamentals are the same.

The divergence may also vary according to where the person is looking. The eyes tend to straighten for close-up sight, but the outward turn is often worse when distance vision is attempted. This underscores the relationship to the adaptation that causes myopia. The patient with either of these symptoms may be striving to function well at close work, and therefore makes sacrifices in his distance vision. In that case, he is apt to be a fair achiever, though seldom more than that.

It is not uncommon for divergent strabismus to show up at one other time of life—as an ultimate adaptation to "middle-aged sight." In that case, it is the end result of continuously using "crutch" lenses to read. When persons who begin to have trouble with close work are given unduly strong reading lenses so that they can see even the smallest type, and when they use them a great deal, the visual system's protest against this unnatural situation may result in an eye turning outward.

Not all problems of divergence are induced by stress, however. In some cases, especially those that show up in the preschool years, we have to be alert to the chance that there is an organic reason—either a congenital defect or the result of an accident. Very infrequently, it can be a problem of faulty motor development, but in that case it would have come from a much more serious interference with growth than the kind of restraints that cause the eyes to cross *inward*. Only a *very* severe restriction, such as the unwise use of a metal foot brace to straighten a turned foot, has been known to distort the child's over-all development enough to bring on this kind of reaction. When things like this are attempted—and sometimes they must be—the parents and doctors should always bear in mind the fact that stress affects the whole body. You cannot just twist this leg, this group of bones and muscles, and expect everything else to stay as it is, any more than you can carelessly manipulate the roots of a plant and expect the stems and leaves to stay unaffected. It is essential to be alert to the possible visual effects and try to compensate by arranging for an especially rich variety of experiences at times when the restraint is not in use.

Whenever I see a case of divergent strabismus at preschool age, I advise that a neurological examination be made at once. This resolves the question of whether any brain damage could be involved. It also tells us what results can be expected from a visual-training program. And it sometimes indicates that a team approach is needed—combining the pediatrician, neurologist, vision specialist, and perhaps a psychologist. Which one will head the team depends on what the problem proves to be—what form of treatment must take priority.

To understand why an eye may turn outward very early in life, keep in mind that visual development goes along with development of the whole neuromuscular system. Like the eyes, this system is divided into two halves. Scientists who have carefully studied a normal child's way of developing find that he first builds a certain skill on one side, then works on the other side for a bit, then merges the two so that he can do the operation with both sides at once. But at some points in this pendulum-style swing, there are times when one side pushes well ahead of the other—resulting in the phenomenon of "handedness," making almost everyone better with either the right or the left side.

In persons who have one eye turning outward and vision in it partly suppressed, we usually find that this side of the body is also less developed than the other. If weighed on two scales—with a foot on each—this side will weigh less. The muscles are less developed on that entire side. Sometimes, this person will have established similar skills with each side, but will not have reached the point of putting the two halves together. Perhaps he can reach out and touch a ball accurately with either hand, but cannot do it smoothly with both hands at once. If this awkwardness exists in the muscles, how obvious it is that the visual system must become involved—for this is the most complex and most delicate part of the body. It is the only place in which both the voluntary and involuntary nervous systems meet. And each eye, although governed mainly by the opposite side of the brain, has connections with both sides of the brain. There is nothing else like it!

CHAPTER 14

Are Nearsighted People Born or Made?

About 25 per cent of the American people are myopic, to judge from my own practice and estimates I have put together from other sources. Many of these persons see well enough near at hand, but details a few feet away may look fuzzy. And at greater distances they miss many things that normally should be seen and enjoyed. The great majority of these people are suffering needlessly— suffering from the effects of pressures that were thrust on them sometime before their twentieth year.

There are those who still insist that this nearsightedness is caused by a defect in the shape of the eyeball. The long-held belief was that the eye is much like a camera, and that an overly long eyeball or improperly shaped cornea would cause the light falling on the retina to be blurred. It was felt that this defect was related to a person's growth, and this seemed to be confirmed by the fact that myopia often did stop progressing between ages sixteen and eighteen. The fact that this also coincided with the school years at a time when few youngsters went beyond the tenth or twelfth grade was not considered.

We can now see that the onset of myopia is much more

closely related to the pattern of educational and working stresses than to physical growth. As a matter of fact, there is increasing research evidence that the eyeballs reach full size by age four and one-half; they do not keep growing through the teen years along with other parts of the body. It is the *functioning* of the system, the way it is used, rather than any defect in it, that causes the nearsighted symptom.

And note that this is a *symptom*. Myopia is not an ailment. It is some people's way of adapting to circumstances that challenge the visual system. There are any number of examples to prove this. One of the most striking is the experience with nuclear submarines that stay under water for very long periods of time. Living in cramped quarters, having little amusement other than reading, many crew members who start out with no apparent visual problem return from a cruise with pronounced nearsightedness. In the face of such evidence, there is no more room for the old notion that vision cannot be changed by environment.

The same statement can be made about astigmatism. This distortion of vision, which may make things appear to be either elongated or stretched sidewise, cannot be explained by the neat mechanical theory that used to be standard: that is, that an imperfection in the curvature of the lens or cornea causes an imperfect image to fall on the retina. The fact is that astigmatism sometimes varies during very short periods of time—worsening dramatically during great tension or an illness, then easing off. Even the direction of the distortion has been known to change completely—from vertical to horizontal. Astigmatism, we now know, is just one more adaptation to environment, and a particularly subtle one.

Instances of defective eyeballs do exist, just as there are congenital defects in other parts of the body. But these are quite rare. As I have mentioned in the last chapter, genetic defects hardly ever occur singly. Anyone born with a real defect is apt to have other structural anomalies. The prevalent nearsightedness we see all around us among completely normal persons is a totally different category of problem.

It should be said, for the sake of completeness, that inherited characteristics do possibly play a part in many cases of myopia—but seldom in the sense of "defects." When we see a family whose members are all myopic, it may well be that they share a common genetic tendency to *adapt* to stress by shifting into nearsighted habits. What would be inherited in that case is not the myopia, but the way of responding to certain challenges. Many inherited tendencies can be turned into constructive channels if they are handled properly. So even if some persons do inherit a tendency to myopia—which is by no means clear—our ability to prevent it from materializing is beyond doubt.

One thing we can be sure of is that we are dealing mainly with persons who are born with perfectly healthy eyes—normal equipment. Some of these persons develop myopia as a result of developmental interference during their very early years—the kind of environmental restraints or deprivation that I have described in discussing other forms of unfavorable adaptation. But the vast majority of nearsightedness results from stress that occurs at the ages emphasized in the chapter called "The Special Cautions"—seven, thirteen to fifteen, and seventeen to twenty. It results from the stress of close work, sometimes combined with internal stresses that occur at climactic times in the process of growing up.

Of course, the individual differences among people make each case unique, so you will realize that I am oversimplifying on purpose. The optometrist has to analyze each patient with great care to avoid being misled by sweeping generalities. But there are some broad general types of case histories which most nearsighted persons share, and it will help your understanding to hear about two people who are representative of a great many others.

Betty C. got her first prescription for glasses in the fourth grade, when a Snellen chart test showed that her visual acuity was poorer than 20/20. This came as a surprise because she had thought she could see all right. Always a bright student, she sat in the front of the classroom and saw the board without difficulty. The glasses did seem to make things look sharper after she got used to them, but they had to be changed many times. The eye doctor gave a new prescription for stronger lenses as often as every year; one of them, in fact, came only six months after an earlier change.

When Betty became a teen-ager and more conscious of herself she often went without her glasses in social situations. It was a visual struggle, but vanity won out. She continues to do without her glasses most of the time. Habit forces her to put them on for close work—reading or sewing—and sometimes she is aware that the eyes begin

to seem tired under those conditions. In fact, she finds
that removing the glasses for a while is refreshing. Since
the glasses are adjusted for distance vision, they are
really too strong for this near-point work, but she has
never questioned the doctor. She has just learned to live
with a world that is never quite comfortable visually.

Unlike Betty's "primary myopia," which became an
overt symptom early in life, my other example's nearsightedness is "secondary." His long-standing visual interference didn't show up until he ran into extra stresses
in college:

Robert M. had always done well in school. His IQ was
quite high and his family was a cultured one, exposing
him to a broad range of interests and wide vocabulary. So
he found himself somewhat ahead of many other children in general knowledge. This head start gave him a
feeling of confidence in the early grades. When he got to
junior high and high school, it helped him to excel in
class discussions. Bob also liked sports and played a lot
of baseball; his hitting was not as steady as he would
have liked, but he was a good enough infielder to be
picked whenever the boys chose up sides. Only one sign
of future trouble might have been spotted if today's
knowledge of vision had existed at that time: Bob tended
to shirk his reading assignments. When he sat with a text-
book before him, he often became sleepy, and very little
of the subject matter stayed with him. But Bob was a
good "audile learner" (learning through listening), and
this earned him better-than-average grades. When his
eyes were screened, he scored a "perfect 20/20" on the
Snellen chart test. So the interference that made close

work and visual learning hard for him was not even suspected.

Then Bob M. went to college—away from home—and suddenly he felt vaguely unsure of himself and off balance. He wasn't getting the hang of his subjects. His early quiz grades were poor. What had happened to Bob was this: At the very time that the challenge of proving himself in new surroundings was putting him under extra pressure, his old way of absorbing information failed him. Learning mainly by ear didn't work at the college level. The tremendous reading load had to be coped with. Bob applied himself to it, but found that the information didn't stay in his head. He had to reread laboriously, trying to organize and remember the facts obtained in this unfamiliar way.

Being determined, more apt to meet challenges than to dodge them, Bob was not one of those who went to pieces. Instead, without understanding his uneasiness, he buckled down harder. He studied longer than he had ever done before. And he did make the grade. He conquered the hard new subjects, the unfamiliar environment, and the abnormally long reading schedule. But this was a new high level of energy demand on his body, so something had to be sacrificed. Bob M. sacrificed the luxury of near- and far-point focusing. Like a tired man who slumps into a soft chair, Bob's tired mind let his eyes slump into the set position that was most needed—a thick-lensed short focus for reading. Bob adapted to the stress. When he noticed that distance vision was impaired, he went to an eye doctor who handed him the usual glasses with minus lenses that allowed his own eyes to slouch even more. From then on, a success in college and in life, Bob kept seeing the easy way—with a visual system geared mainly to close work. Now, with the first signs of middle-aged sight, he is aware that his near-point vision is becoming a problem, too.

Please don't read any unintended precepts into this example. I don't mean it to indicate that Bob's younger school days should have been arranged differently or that going away to college is any more of a risk than staying near home. Stress may occur in any human situation. Avoiding it entirely is not a practical response to the challenge of life. My point is that today we could recognize such a young person's visual interference quickly and prescribe counterstress lenses or training to keep it from becoming a problem. By making close work easier and more productive from the early school years on, we prepare the system to move through high-pressure periods easily and without reliance on crutch-type eyeglasses.

While the experiences of Betty C. and Robert M. are only two out of thousands of possible variations, they illustrate the general principle that causes and perpetuates most cases of nearsightedness.

Just how "bad" myopia is depends on how it affects a person's life. For example, a very bookish individual who wants to spend his life as a researcher and cares hardly at all for distance vision is really adapting to his career if he becomes nearsighted. Some company employment managers finally learned a few years ago that they were turning away their best applicants when they insisted on ordinary eye acuity tests for jobs that involved assem-

bling delicate instruments and small electronic compo-
nents. Many of the persons selected did poor work, grew
irritable, or developed headaches. When myopic persons
were hired, they raised the efficiency markedly. For this
reason, I never tell a patient that he should take training or wear special lenses to try to get rid of myopia. If
his myopia is causing him problems in his life, then, yes—
we should try to treat it.

The old approach is to prescribe minus lenses, which
will distort sizes and distances, thereby causing the patient to make inward adjustments to compensate for the
distortions.

A less destructive approach taken in recent years is
to give a prescription that "undercorrects" somewhat, that
is, glasses that provide a little less than perfect sharpness
of sight at twenty feet or more. Since these create less
distortion of reality and are less of a crutch, they cause
less inner damage. But clearly, this concept of merely re-
ducing the harmfulness is not very satisfying in a dynamic age.

Our modern approach is to let the patient know that
actual improvement is available through a combination
of lenses and visual training. The lenses are primarily for
close work, for this is where the stresses occur—the
stresses that caused the myopia to begin with. If the condition is such that some help for distance vision is essential, we suggest bifocals in order to be sure that just
the right lens is in front of the eye for both near and
far points. And if the patient seems to be one who is
motivated to work for improvement, we may suggest
visual training to *learn* how to see better.

Bear in mind that myopia is learned to begin with. It is a habit of overfocusing—sometimes practiced to the point of creating mechanical changes in the system, sometimes not. This habit is made a part of one's way of life, in order to cope with some difficulty or challenge. We can often recommend ways to change the environmental conditions and then relearn the visual process on a nonmyopic basis. The degree of success depends on how firmly the problem is fixed into the system, how motivated the person is to work for improvement, and what the conditions of his life are.

A great deal of myopia research is under way, along many lines. There is experimentation with drugs put into the eyes. There are laboratory studies of the effects of bright or dim light on myopia. And there is a great deal of research on the relationship of diet and general health to the problem of nearsightedness. Much of this is to the good. Vision, being the most complex of all human functions, cannot fail to be much influenced by everything that affects the body's health. But because myopia is a habit, it is inescapable that breaking that habit and relearning a healthier one must be the principal avenue to solid improvement.

CHAPTER 15

The Double Meaning of "Farsightedness"

Farsightedness is not—although every layman very reasonably assumes it is—the opposite of nearsightedness. In fact, this term, which is technically known as *hyperopia*, describes two entirely separate conditions—one of which is very favorable, the other distinctly troublesome. I'll try to clarify this unfortunate terminology in a brief way, even at the risk of oversimplifying somewhat.

Hyperopia doesn't refer to how *far* a person sees. It means *flexibility*—the ability to keep seeing well even when an obstacle or stress tends to diminish the normal sharpness of his sight.

When an optometrist tests for hyperopia he measures the ability to maintain 20/20 acuity even when looking through plus lenses—the lenses normally used for near-point work. This ability, in itself, does not indicate a problem, although some practitioners still mistakenly treat it as such. On the contrary, if there are no complicating factors, the ability to adapt and overcome such an obstacle is a margin of safety to cope with the varying degrees of stress that will be met. When a challenging situation temporarily reduces the range of vision—an accident on the road ahead, a ball coming swiftly from the far court, a friend signaling from a distance—the person with this kind of "farsightedness" still has enough bounce in his visual system to see adequately.

Man developed this flexibility while still in a primitive state. If our early ancestor had lacked it, the stress caused by catching sight of a saber-toothed tiger would have turned him momentarily myopic and led to a quick end. But the adjustability of his system left him with sharp-enough sight to aim his spear.

This was *transient* stress, and the system quickly returned to normal. Modern man is having to handle a kind of *persistent* stress that even his fairly recent ancestors seldom had to reckon with—the demand for near-point vision over long periods of time. The two eyes turn inward to point at the object, the pupils contract, the lenses adjust to distribute light onto the retinas in a new pattern that the brain can interpret.

In order to be ready for these coming near-point stresses and yet not lose his distance vision, a child should have developed slight hyperopia by the time he is about six; if not, we know that his system is not flexible enough, and we can predict that he will eventually become near-sighted under stress or will slacken his visual efficiency and be less successful in his studies. He is walking a tight-rope. The child with normal hyperopia is walking on a broad path that allows room for a more relaxed trip through life.

There is another condition commonly mislabeled with the same term—"farsightedness." We distinguish it by the name *adverse hyperopia*. This means that the person has below-average range of ability to adjust to various visual demands, particularly at the near point. When the visual challenge is accompanied by stress, the range narrows even further.

This condition is a particularly urgent sign that developmental help or other training is needed. For much of modern living does involve near-point vision. And although compensatory lenses can be prescribed for adverse farsightedness, they are not an answer because they further lessen the "degree of freedom" that the person had. They can only lead to a need for increasingly powerful glasses.

When we see a very high degree of adverse hyperopia we have to check the possibility that some pathological condition may exist. Some cases of mental retardation are accompanied by "farsightedness"; and this can be a vicious cycle, since the scarcity of good visual information will, in turn, handicap the mind's development. There are also cases that result from serious illness and high fever. And environmental factors may occasionally be to blame: Poor diets and lack of mental stimulation in the very early years, for instance, can permanently stunt the mind and the visual system. But these are not the common causes of adverse hyperopia.

Most of it results from adaptation to inappropriate lenses.

Normal hyperopia can be turned into the pernicious variety by improper eyeglasses. Tragically, these are sometimes prescribed for children whose farsightedness is of the favorable, necessary kind. Practitioners unfamiliar with the modern functional approach notice the hyperopic measurement and suggest glasses that take over the focusing. They gradually rob the system of that ability—absorb part of its range. So they create adverse hyperopia.

This same chain of events is also seen in persons who are encountering the problem of middle-aged sight. The right counterstress lenses can actually assist in preserving good vision at near and far points, as we'll see in the next chapter. But glasses that ignore the function of the entire system—that aim only to make the tiniest print legible—can be very destructive.

To sum up: Farsightedness is a misleading term because it means two different things and neither of them is the opposite of nearsightedness. It has nothing to do with seeing too far. People who do see beyond the 20/20 level of acuity may or may not be "farsighted," in the problem sense. The real question involved is *range* of vision. If the wrong lenses take over a part of this normal span, they will diminish it. Lenses properly used can protect and preserve the ability to adjust to all distances— which is as necessary to comfortable living as a good range of high and low notes is to a singer's voice.

CHAPTER 16

Get More Out of Golf, Tennis, Dancing

A few years ago the Cincinnati Reds baseball team called in an optometrist, Dr. Bruce Wolff, to give the players visual training. It was unusual, but it made as much sense as calling in a pitching coach or a consultant on hitting, because total vision is really what sports are all about. In our work we always talk about hand-and-eye activities —meaning the interplay between seeing, calculating, and then acting.

Vision care cannot teach you to play a game, but it can create abilities and freedom of action that will very much enhance sports performance. The reverse also is true: Taking part in sports is a very effective way to build many visual skills, especially if the person has learned some of the principles of vision and consciously applies them on the playing field.

If you happen to have the co-ordination of a Willie Mays, who can catch his falling hat with one hand while grabbing a fly ball with the other, there's probably nothing we could teach you about hand-and-eye movements. But almost everybody, including quite good athletes, is pretty limited in those "degrees of freedom" that I mentioned earlier. If several things happen at once, we say that we got "flustered," meaning that our nervous system didn't have the freedom to cope with several actions at the same time. It's somewhat comparable to an old-fashioned telephone cable that could handle only a few calls at a time; as modern, coaxial cables developed, the same system could handle much more activity with great ease. We'd all like to move in that direction if we could, to do more with less strain.

So quite a few men have come to me, and I know that many other optometrists have had the same experience, and asked, "Could any of these methods you use improve my golf game?" The answer to that is yes. My job in that case is to improve the over-all relationship of the visual and muscular systems so that the man becomes, in a general sense, a "better athlete." His golf game is bound to benefit. Of course, as his golf improves, his vision and bodily condition will benefit, too.

The simple act of swinging a club in such a way as to make a little golf ball fly in just a certain path is really a perfect example of why vision is a head-to-toe matter. If you have tried it, you know that awkward feeling of first standing up at a tee and suddenly becoming conscious of how unsure your balance is. A moment ago you were walking along and feeling completely in balance. Now you can't quite decide where this foot should be, how far from the ball you should stand, what path the club head should follow as you draw it back. Why all the doubts? Because the brain is trying to compute a lot of new information that is coming in from all the sensory systems: the eyes reporting on the location of the hole, the fairway, the traps, ball, and club head; the sense of touch indicating what each part of the body is doing, signaling the lay of the land beneath the feet, informing about the club's weight and the path it takes as the back-swing begins; touch and hearing together sending word about wind direction. This is a highly oversimplified ac-count of the inpouring of data to the brain, in the form of electrical impulses. The various bits of information have to be compared with each other. And more than that, they have to be matched against past experience that is filed away in the brain. Based on all this, the computer makes a series of decisions, sending instruc-tions to the muscles in your ankles, knees, hips, shoulders, elbows, wrists, and fingers in order to create the swing that your mind envisions.

Many golf pros recommend a process of conscious visu-alizing—picturing in advance the path of the club head and later the trajectory you hope the ball will follow. But in fact, every act we do is performed *mentally* before we order the muscles to go through with it. Depending on the degree of skill or the difficulty of the task, we may do this very slowly and deliberately or with almost no delay.

What happens in visual training that helps a person to do this? The trainee learns to be conscious of vision, just as he must be in any sports situation. He uses his eyes more alertly, feeds information with more precision into his mental computer, and relates his muscle move-ments more exactly to the conclusions his mind has reached.

Take this standard training procedure as an example:

A trainee walks along a narrow beam, just a couple of inches off the floor, but forcing him to balance, and he keeps his eyes fixed on a rotating colored disk set at eye level in front of him. Coming forward to the front end of the beam is not too difficult; retracing his steps backward without losing balance and without taking his eye off the turning disk is harder. With practice he learns to visualize the length of that beam more accurately, to have a clearer mental idea of how long his steps are, so that even when walking backward he knows when he is nearing the end of the beam. He is developing the freedom to compute many situations at once and to relate them all to each other, forming a smooth, unified flow of action. I needn't explain to you why this person will later step up to a golf ball with better balance and more confidence in his ability to swing smoothly and surely.

Tennis is another sport that is directly related to visual training. In fact, the game itself is one of the most thorough forms of visual training I can imagine. It demands quick changes of focus from far to near points, lightning-fast perception of where the ball will land, computation of how high it will bounce, and multiple decisions about how to strike the ball so that it will follow a mentally envisioned path and elude an opponent who is seen peripherally.

But let me caution that piddling haphazardly at a sport is not a way of getting these benefits to the system. Doing things poorly in such games as golf and tennis is frustrating and, in my own opinion, actually harmful. Any form of repeated failure is bad for the mind and nervous sys-

tem, just as success is good for us. And this is not just a
vague psychological matter of confidence. There are hard
reasons behind it. Every action we make is stored in the
brain as past experience. An error that is analyzed and
understood can have positive value. But haphazard and
repeated errors are destructive. A boy who runs clumsily
after a tennis ball, swings an improperly-held racket, and
knocks the ball into the net may be "getting good exercise
anyway" in the view of some. But I think he is building a
lot of bad habits into his system. Trying to record the results of that last try, his mind can only become more confused. Unless it is a remarkably agile mind to begin with,
how can it possibly get good corrective information from
this mass of mistakes? The boy will tighten up, grip his
racket harder, swing more hesitantly. Even when he happens to hit a good shot, he won't know why.

One of the principles of all learning is: Practice in the
way you wish ultimately to perform. Learn from error
—but never practice an error.

So start any sport with good professional instruction
—that's my advice. The notion of "just having fun" at a
sport without bothering to do it well is a myth. The
smoother your movements and the better your results,
the greater the fun. And that habit of doing things well
will carry over into other aspects of life.

Dancing is another pleasurable activity that is related
to this whole subject. In most offices where visual training is given, you will see a simple device that we call
a "Marsden ball"—a white rubber ball about the size of
a softball that is suspended by a cord from the ceiling

so that it hangs to a little below the eye level of the person using it. Printed letters and numbers—in differing sizes and at odd angles—are marked all over the ball with a marking pencil. Many different exercises can be done with this ball, some of them very sophisticated and requiring professional equipment. But one routine is so simple that anyone can do it at home. The object is to set the ball swaying in an oval or circular motion and then to follow it with two pointers held in the hands. Two long lead pencils will do, although long plastic sticks sold in toy departments are preferable. This is very hard to do at

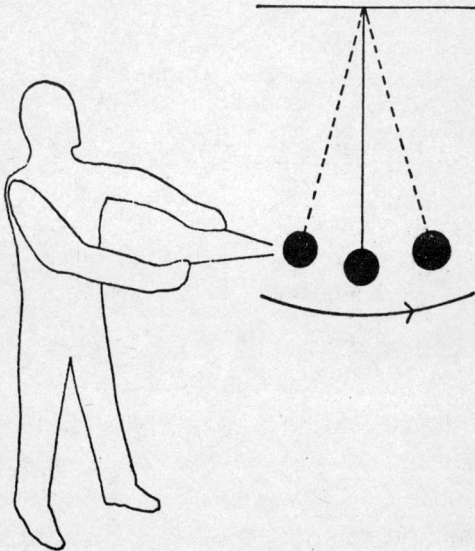

Patient following Marsden ball accurately with two pointers.

first. When told to look for a certain letter and then to hold the pointers as near as possible to that letter while the ball makes five complete orbits, the beginner will usually move about clumsily, then hold the pointer ends six or eight inches from the ball and only half-follow it with jerky movements. But after a time every earnest trainee improves greatly at it, which means that the eyes and the whole co-ordinative system right down to the balls of the feet are working at a higher level of harmony.

One of my colleagues told me that one of the young girls taking training in his office moved so gracefully in following the Marsden ball, stepping so lightly and keeping the pointers within half an inch of the selected point, that he remarked aloud, "This is like watching a ballerina." The swaying girl heard him and said, "As a matter of fact, I've been doing much better at my ballet lessons since I started visual training."

These practical results give the optometrist even more satisfaction than his own professional assessment of the patient's progress. Visual care is not an end in itself. It is a doorway, opening on to new activities, skills, pleasures. No goals that we can set for the patient are as meaningful as his own aspirations. So our criterion of success is the patient's own report that he is now doing the things he had always hoped to do.

CHAPTER 17

Must Age Harm Your Vision?

Those fortyish persons who have to hold the phone book farther away and have trouble reading the menu in a restaurant may feel better to know that they are suffering from a teen-age development. The process leading to presbyopia or middle-aged sight begins around age thirteen.

That may make it seem that such an inevitable decline is not worth trying to prevent. But the truth is that we can do a lot of things to stall off the problem aspect of it and to limit the extent of its bother. It's like any other aspect of aging. We all *want* to grow older in years, since the alternative is not generally appealing. And we know that the process of living involves constant tissue changes in our bodies. But what a difference it makes whether we keep in the best possible shape or not! Compare the dancer who still moves lightly and gracefully as he approaches seventy with the out-of-shape suburbanite who is a quarter-century younger but can barely plod his way around a golf course. Maybe they were born with different characteristics; but nobody doubts that their ways of life have a lot to do with their differences.

So it is with the eyes. We can get very different results from them for very much longer, depending on how we treat them—and despite the fact that many internal changes are going on.

The reason that age affects vision is worth understanding. Your eyes are governed by both nervous systems— the only part of the body that has this complexity, by the way. The *voluntary* nervous system moves the entire eyeball, so that you can consciously point your eyes wherever you wish. The *involuntary* nervous system controls the focusing without your realizing it. These two sources of guidance learn to co-operate in what is called a "patterned relationship." But this pattern has in it enough freedom to work serviceably even when the two systems get somewhat out of step, as they do.

It is the *difference* in the aging of the two systems that eventually creates a problem. The voluntary one declines only very slowly throughout your life; but the involuntary system drops off more steeply in its activity —beginning in the early teen years. The gap goes on growing for about twenty-five years without being noticeable, but at a certain point—usually in the mid-thirties —it begins to cause small troubles. The first of these are not usually accompanied by difficulty in seeing. They take the form of discomfort and lower efficiency—reduced reading speed, more errors in typing or addition, poorer golf scores, and so on.

At some point the gap between the two systems produces a symptom that cannot be mistaken. When a person can voluntarily point his eyes at anything he likes —as near as he likes—but the involuntary muscles don't respond enough to create a familiar light pattern, a stress is set up in the mind and body. The brain gets conflicting information that it has to translate as a blur. It signals the whole system to try harder, racing the engine, and the stress in itself does further damage to the involuntary nervous apparatus. Whereas it had declined slowly in all the earlier years, it now takes a real nose dive, urgently sending the person to an eye doctor for reading glasses.

Now comes the question: Can this be prevented? As of now, the answer is no, we don't know any way to avoid the process entirely. We do, however, have a way of minimizing it. This consists of watching carefully to anticipate the time when the divergence of the two systems will become a threat—*before* it is noticeable to the patient. If the optometrist can identify this early presbyopia before it begins to put stress on the seeing system, he prescribes reading lenses that can really be called preventive glasses. We cannot stop the normal physiological changes, but we prevent the maladaptations that multiply the ills.

This is a totally different principle from waiting until there is noticeable trouble in reading and then putting on lenses that magnify the print and take over all the focusing job. These encourage adverse adaptations in the body. They can only lead to further decline, so that many a person over forty gets stronger glasses year after year. They rob the system of its range—its freedom to focus—so that distance vision becomes affected, too, even in persons who never had a trace of that problem.

The counterstress lenses we now prescribe for near

work restore a more appropriate relationship between the two nervous systems. These can often be small half-eye lenses or bifocals with just plain glass in the upper part. If preferred, they can be full-size lenses, but should be slipped off the moment that close work is interrupted, so that the eyes are not seeing through a lens for anything but close work.

With this most modern approach we find that the need for lens changes is much less frequent.

There are some who say, "If I have to wear glasses anyway, what's the difference exactly how strong the lenses are?" They should realize, for one thing, that it is going to make quite a difference if they are lucky enough to live into their seventies, eighties, and beyond, as more people are doing these days. At that point, they are likely to need very heavy glasses, and possibly even a big magnifying glass, as well, to painfully read a newspaper; while the person who had the more advanced type of care will simply slip on a pair of ordinary glasses and live a full life, indoors and out.

Even in the shorter run, it should make a lot of difference to us how strong our glasses have to be and whether they are being changed often. Our eyes mirror the condition of the entire body. If we are preventing stress well enough to keep the two nervous systems operating at a relatively high level, we are actually aging much more slowly than someone else of the same calendar age whose vision is continually slipping.

Beyond this one limited subject of presbyopia, it is absolutely not true that age makes it impossible to overcome other visual problems. With the proper attitude and care, one can reap the benefits of being older, rather than being stymied by the fact. Anything that children can accomplish, adults can usually do even better. They are more highly motivated, because they fully appreciate the disadvantages of not seeing perfectly. They can understand what the doctor is asking of them, and they can frequently suggest adjustments in method that are a genuine improvement. (I wish more doctors would listen to the suggestions made by their patients—although they are usually made hesitantly, for fear the doctor will take offense. Many techniques that I am now using in visual training have been improved and refined by applying the comments made by patients.)

It is generally supposed that cross-eyes, for example, must be cured in childhood or it will be too late. But when adults do come to take visual training for this defect, they usually learn the knack of straightening the eyes faster than children do. The same is true of adults with a "lazy eye" that has been left idling all their lives. In cases where they are forced to improve that eye, they make surprisingly fast progress.

Many adults also come to the vision specialist with a problem very similar to that of the school-age underachievers—and they, too, get fine results. These are persons whose eye measurements seem all right, but who simply cannot enjoy or profit from their reading. Even persons around retirement age are included in this category. I recall that one retired admiral came to me feeling quite low because the dream he had nurtured for years while waiting to retire had gone sour. He had accumulated a great library of books that he had never had time to read. His big wish was to spend days of quietly reading and enjoying all these works. Six months earlier his retirement had come through, and now here he was, saying, "I find that I can't really read for long." Why not? "Well, I get headaches, or I become very sleepy—no matter how interesting the subject is to me. The job of reading just seems to spoil all my pleasure in the contents of the book." This man, with the glasses he was wearing, had perfectly good "eyesight." But his visual system was tuned to the reading of short memos and then hours spent in conferences and briefing rooms; it just wasn't keyed to long reading. He took visual training directed straight at his particular goals, and in a very few months he was completely happy.

I have had a number of other retired patients with similar ambitions. It is surprising how many persons have a yen to improve themselves through reading after they retire. Some even want to read through an entire encyclopedia! Such persons—whether we happen to agree with their goals or not—are even more likely than children to achieve full success, because they know exactly what they want.

I'd like to stress that the chance of visual improvement is available to anyone at any age. It may not always lead to getting rid of eyeglasses or to changes in the measurements of the eye. It *can* lead to the real purpose of vision: a more effective person who is better co-ordinated, better equipped to reach his own goals. Sometimes those goals change in the course of living, and the person wants to tune his visual abilities to still another pitch. I am usually heartened when I see this because a person who is still growing and developing is always younger than his years. In nature nothing can be static. If you try to stay exactly where you were, you lose ground. The only way to hold your own against time is by taking the offensive—determining to keep making improvements.

All that we have been saying about vision—at home, at work, in school—relates very closely to the old question of whether each of us is the product of heredity or environment. There is no longer any doubt that we are both. We are what we were at birth plus all that we have seen and felt and thought since then. But the awareness of how greatly vision shapes the product can make us all a little less content to accept mediocrity with resignation.

In an era when parents and educators sometimes wonder about the importance of their own roles, the lesson of vision is worth pondering. Every small detail in a child's living and studying arrangements has a formative effect on how he will perceive, what the world will seem like inside his head, what future acts his life will consist of as a result.

And this applies to your own future as well. Your visual system is not a finished product just because you are grown. It is flexible, dynamic, ever evolving. Part of its future is rooted in the past. But a big part is still up to you.

Index

Accidents, 94

Achievement, 16–17, 20, 46–49, 51, 56 ff; reading and, 51, 56 ff, 72 ff; and school environment, 67–68

Achievement Center for Children, 48

Adaptation, 4, 12, 29, 119; astigmatism and, 99; myopia and, 98, 103; strabismus and, 86, 92, 93; stress and, 73, 80, 81, 108

Adverse hyperopia, 107–9

Age (aging), and vision, 117–23

Alexander, E. B., v, 14

Alternate wink exercise, 33–34

Amblyopia, 42

American Optometric Association, 21, 49

"Angels in the Snow," (game), 48

"Annapolis Syndrome," 76

Arithmetic, 46

Astigmatism, 98–99

Athletics, 110–14

Auditory learners, 74, 101

Babies, 40–49, 72; and learning and role of parents, 40–49, 72; and strabismus, 84–91

Balance, 2, 3, 70, 111. See also Imbalance

"Balance board," construction and use of, 32–33, 34, 37

Balloons, 44

Balls, use in learning and training, 18, 44, 61, 114–16

Barstow, Ralph, v

Bates, Dr., and "sight without glasses," 6–7

Becker School, 67–68

Bed, reading in, 27–28

Bifocals, 6, 11–12, 90, 104, 120

Blocks, infant learning and, 41, 44

Blue collar workers, 75

Blurring, 19, 73, 97, 119

Body movements, vision and, 19–20, 42–43

Brain, the, 3, 5, 16, 112, 119; posture and, 28; strabismus and, 84, 95, 96; vision primarily in, 2, 3

Breathing exercise, 32–33

"Brightness factors," 24

Camera, analogy of eyes to, 4, 97

Card games, 37

Ceilings, 24, 37–38

Chairs, vision and, 26, 42–43, 66

Children, xiv, 7–12, 25, 29, 36, 40–49, 64–69, 70, 71, 78–91 ff, 123; achievement and vision in (See Achievement); home environment and, 25, 26–27, 40–49; myopic, 9–12, 70, 72–76, 79–80, 97 ff; parents and, 40–49; and reading, 50–55, 56–63 (See also Reading); and school environment, 64–69 (See also Schools; and studying and vision, 56–63; and visual problems, 70, 71–76 (See also specific aspects, problems); and visual training, 15–17 (See also Visual training)

Closed-eye fixations, 35

Closed-eye rotations, 34

Close work, (close-up work). See Near-point vision (near-point concentration)

Genes (genetics). *See* Heredity
Georgetown University, 54
Gesell, Arnold, xii, 72
Gesell Institute of Child Development, 48
Getman, G. N., 49
Glare, 23, 29, 66
Golf, 111–12, 113
Greenstein, Tole, 64

Habits, visual, 22, 84, 105, 114
Hand-and-eye activities, 110
"Handedness", 58, 62, 96
Harmon, Darell Boyd, vi, 66
Headaches, 3, 73
Head rotations, 34–35
Head-to-toe vision, 3, 111
Hearing, sense of, 2, 74, 101, 112
Hemingway, Ernest, 52
Heredity (hereditary influences; inheritance), 1, 4, 58, 83, 123; myopia and, 9, 99; visual training and, 17, 58
Home environment, 22, 30, 84 ff; visual training and, 31–39, 59
Homework, regulation of, 68
How to Develop Your Child's Intelligence, 49
Huxley, Aldous, 52
Hyperopia, 106–9

Illness, 28, 68, 71, 78, 98, 108. *See also* Disease
Imbalance, visual, 42, 83
Indirect Lighting, 25
Infants. *See* Babies
Information (knowledge), 80, 82, 112; eyes as source of brain's, 2, 5; strabismus and, 84 ff; visual training and, 16–21
Inheritance. *See* Heredity
Intelligence, development in young children, 40–49. *See also* Information; Learning; specific aspects
Involuntary nervous system, 118–20
Inward-turning eyes, 82–91

Journal of Ophthalmology, 76

Kephart, Newell C., 45–46, 49
Kindergarten, 58

Lamps, 23, 24–25
Language, 60
Learning, 80, 114 (*See also* Information; Intelligence; Schools); reading and, 50–55, 56–63, 72 ff; readiness for, 58–59; schools and vision, 65, 66, 70, 71–76; visual training and, 18, 36 (*See also* Visual training); in young children, 40–49
Left and right direction, 58, 62, 96
Lens, human, 4, 98
Lenses (eyeglasses), 8–9, 12, 28–29, 54, 57, 89, 103, 109, 119 (*See also* specific kinds); and aging, 119–22; developmental, 8, 9; and hyperopia, 108–9; and myopia, 103–4; preventive, 7, 8–9, 11, 12, 119; purpose of, 6–13; sight without, 6–7; and strabismus, 83, 89, 90, 92–93; and visual training, 17, 20, 89 (*See also* Visual training)
Light (lights; lighting), 4; at home, 23–25, 28–29, 30; and infants, 40, 41; and myopia, 105; at school, 65–66
Light-diffusers, 65
Locke, John, 69

Marsden ball, 114–16
Mays, Willie, 110
Mental retardation, 108
Metronome, use of, 20, 34, 35
Middle-aged sight. *See* Presbyopia
Minus lenses, 10–11, 92–93, 104
"Missing the Ceiling" (game), 37–38
Mobiles, use of, 41
Mommy and Daddy—You Can Help Me Learn to See, 49
Motivation, 17–18, 92, 104, 105, 121

Right and left directions, 58, 62, 96
Room arrangement, 26, 40, 65
Rotation exercises: closed-eye, 34; head, 34–35; neck, 33; pie-tin, 37

Schools (education): myopia and, 98 ff; reading and, 56–63, 70, 72 ff; safeguarding of vision and, 64–69, 70, 71–76
Seated position, proper, 65, 66
Second graders, 58–59, 62, 72, 93
Selye, Hans, 4
Senses, 2–4, 80, 111–12
Seventeen-to-twenty age group, 74–76, 100
Shapes, and learning, 45, 48, 61, 62
"Sight without glasses," xiv, 6–7, 12–13
Six-to-ten year olds, 8, 72, 74, 100
Skeffington, A. M., vi, 14
Skills, 48, 50–55, 56–63, 72 ff; visual training for, 18–21
Smell, sense of, 2
Space (spatial relations), 42, 43, 45–46, 48, 58–60, 62
Speech, 60
Speed, reading, 54–55; courses in, 54–55
Spelling, 46, 47, 56, 59
Sports, 110–14
Square test, 67
Strabismus, 15, 42; convergent, 82–91, 121; divergent, 92–96
Stress, 2, 4, 5, 8–13, 68, 70 ff, 98 ff, 106 ff; adaptation and, 4, 12, 73, 80, 81, 86, 92 ff, 98 ff; environmental, 23, 24, 26; myopia and, 98–104; special cautions on, 70–77; strabismus and, 86, 92 ff; transient and permanent, 107; visual training and, 16
Study (studying), 56–63, 67, 68, 70–76
Success Through Play, 45–46, 49
Suction-cup rattles, 43
Sunglasses, 29
Sunshine, 28–29
Surgery, 15, 83, 86, 90; "limited," 91
Swinging balls, and visual training, 18
Symbols (symbolizing), 53, 58, 61

Tables, proper height for, 26
Target cards, use of, 33–34, 35
Taste, sense of, 2
Teachers and teaching. *See* Parents; Schools
Teen-agers, 72–73, 119
Television, 25–26, 28, 60
Tennis, 113
Tests, visual, 64–65, 67, 77
Texas schools, 66–68, 72
Three-year-olds, 85–86, 88
Tilted work surfaces, 27
Tilting of head, 70
Touch, sense of, 2, 112
Toys, 41, 43, 44, 89
Training glasses, 20
Tutoring, 57, 59, 63
TV watching, 25–26, 28, 60
20/20 vision, 62, 73, 74, 100, 101

Underachievers, 56, 62, 72 ff
Undercorrection, 104

Visual problems, 57–63 ff; 78–81 ff. *See also* specific aspects, problems
Visual training, 7, 9, 12, 83, 89, 95, 104; aging and, 121–23; avocations and, 110–16; exercises for, 31–39; reading and, 54, 59, 60, 63; what it is, 14–21
Voluntary nervous system, 118–20

Walls, 24, 26
"What Is It? Where Is It?" (game), 36
Winking exercise, 33–34
Wolff, Bruce, 110
Working conditions, 22, 26–27, 30

MELVIN POWERS SELF-IMPROVEMENT LIBRARY

ASTROLOGY

ASTROLOGY: A FASCINATING HISTORY P. Naylor	2.00
ASTROLOGY: HOW TO CHART YOUR HOROSCOPE Max Heindel	2.00
ASTROLOGY: YOUR PERSONAL SUN-SIGN GUIDE Beatrice Ryder	3.00
ASTROLOGY FOR EVERYDAY LIVING Janet Harris	2.00
ASTROLOGY MADE EASY Astarte	2.00
ASTROLOGY MADE PRACTICAL Alexandra Kayhle	2.00
ASTROLOGY, ROMANCE, YOU AND THE STARS Anthony Norvell	3.00
MY WORLD OF ASTROLOGY Sydney Omarr	3.00
THOUGHT DIAL Sydney Omarr	2.00
ZODIAC REVEALED Rupert Gleadow	2.00

BRIDGE & POKER

ADVANCED POKER STRATEGY & WINNING PLAY A. D. Livingston	2.00
BRIDGE BIDDING MADE EASY Edwin Kantar	5.00
BRIDGE CONVENTIONS Edwin Kantar	4.00
COMPLETE DEFENSIVE BRIDGE PLAY Edwin B. Kantar	10.00
HOW TO IMPROVE YOUR BRIDGE Alfred Sheinwold	2.00
HOW TO WIN AT POKER Terence Reese & Anthony T. Watkins	2.00
SECRETS OF WINNING POKER George S. Coffin	3.00
TEST YOUR BRIDGE PLAY Edwin B. Kantar	3.00

BUSINESS STUDY & REFERENCE

CONVERSATION MADE EASY Elliot Russell	2.00
EXAM SECRET Dennis B. Jackson	2.00
FIX-IT BOOK Arthur Symons	2.00
HOW TO DEVELOP A BETTER SPEAKING VOICE M. Hellier	2.00
HOW TO MAKE A FORTUNE IN REAL ESTATE Albert Winnikoff	3.00
HOW TO MAKE MONEY IN REAL ESTATE Stanley L. McMichael	2.00
INCREASE YOUR LEARNING POWER Geoffrey A. Dudley	2.00
MAGIC OF NUMBERS Robert Tocquet	2.00
PRACTICAL GUIDE TO BETTER CONCENTRATION Melvin Powers	2.00
PRACTICAL GUIDE TO PUBLIC SPEAKING Maurice Forley	2.00
7 DAYS TO FASTER READING William S. Schaill	2.00
SONGWRITERS' RHYMING DICTIONARY Jane Shaw Whitfield	3.00
SPELLING MADE EASY Lester D. Basch & Dr. Milton Finkelstein	2.00
STUDENT'S GUIDE TO BETTER GRADES J. A. Rickard	2.00
TEST YOURSELF — Find Your Hidden Talent Jack Shafer	2.00
YOUR WILL & WHAT TO DO ABOUT IT Attorney Samuel G. Kling	2.00

CHESS & CHECKERS

BEGINNER'S GUIDE TO WINNING CHESS Fred Reinfeld	2.00
BETTER CHESS — How to Play Fred Reinfeld	2.00
CHECKERS MADE EASY Tom Wiswell	2.00
CHESS IN TEN EASY LESSONS Larry Evans	2.00
CHESS MADE EASY Milton L. Hanauer	2.00
CHESS MASTERY — A New Approach Fred Reinfeld	2.00
CHESS PROBLEMS FOR BEGINNERS edited by Fred Reinfeld	2.00
CHESS SECRETS REVEALED Fred Reinfeld	2.00
CHESS STRATEGY — An Expert's Guide Fred Reinfeld	2.00
CHESS TACTICS FOR BEGINNERS edited by Fred Reinfeld	2.00
CHESS THEORY & PRACTICE Morry & Mitchell	2.00
HOW TO WIN AT CHECKERS Fred Reinfeld	2.00
1001 BRILLIANT WAYS TO CHECKMATE Fred Reinfeld	2.00
1001 WINNING CHESS SACRIFICES & COMBINATIONS Fred Reinfeld	3.00
SOVIET CHESS Edited by R. G. Wade	3.00

COOKERY & HERBS

CULPEPER'S HERBAL REMEDIES Dr. Nicholas Culpeper	2.00
FAST GOURMET COOKBOOK Poppy Cannon	2.50
HEALING POWER OF HERBS May Bethel	2.00
HERB HANDBOOK Dawn MacLeod	2.00

_____HERBS FOR COOKING AND HEALING *Dr. Donald Law*	2.00
_____HERBS FOR HEALTH How to Grow & Use Them *Louise Evans Doole*	2.00
_____HOME GARDEN COOKBOOK Delicious Natural Food Recipes *Ken Kraft*	3.00
_____MEDICAL HERBALIST *edited by Dr. J. R. Yemm*	3.00
_____NATURAL FOOD COOKBOOK *Dr. Harry C. Bond*	2.00
_____NATURE'S MEDICINES *Richard Lucas*	2.00
_____VEGETABLE GARDENING FOR BEGINNERS *Hugh Wiberg*	2.00
_____VEGETABLES FOR TODAY'S GARDENS *R. Milton Carleton*	2.00
_____VEGETARIAN COOKERY *Janet Walker*	2.00
_____VEGETARIAN COOKING MADE EASY & DELECTABLE *Veronica Vezza*	2.00
_____VEGETARIAN DELIGHTS — A Happy Cookbook for Health *K. R. Mehta*	2.00
_____VEGETARIAN GOURMET COOKBOOK *Joyce McKinnel*	2.00

HEALTH

_____DR. LINDNER'S SPECIAL WEIGHT CONTROL METHOD	1.00
_____HELP YOURSELF TO BETTER SIGHT *Margaret Darst Corbett*	3.00
_____HOW TO IMPROVE YOUR VISION *Dr. Robert A. Kraskin*	2.00
_____HOW YOU CAN STOP SMOKING PERMANENTLY *Ernest Caldwell*	2.00
_____LSD — THE AGE OF MIND *Bernard Roseman*	2.00
_____MIND OVER PLATTER *Peter G. Lindner, M.D.*	2.00
_____NEW CARBOHYDRATE DIET COUNTER *Patti Lopez-Pereira*	1.00
_____PSYCHEDELIC ECSTASY *William Marshall & Gilbert W. Taylor*	2.00
_____YOU CAN LEARN TO RELAX *Dr. Samuel Gutwirth*	2.00
_____YOUR ALLERGY—What To Do About It *Allan Knight, M.D.*	2.00

HOBBIES

_____BEACHCOMBING FOR BEGINNERS *Norman Hickin*	2.00
_____BLACKSTONE'S MODERN CARD TRICKS *Harry Blackstone*	2.00
_____BLACKSTONE'S SECRETS OF MAGIC *Harry Blackstone*	2.00
_____COIN COLLECTING FOR BEGINNERS *Burton Hobson & Fred Reinfeld*	2.00
_____ENTERTAINING WITH ESP *Tony 'Doc' Shiels*	2.00
_____400 FASCINATING MAGIC TRICKS YOU CAN DO *Howard Thurston*	3.00
_____GOULD'S GOLD & SILVER GUIDE TO COINS *Maurice Gould*	2.00
_____HOW I TURN JUNK INTO FUN AND PROFIT *Sari*	3.00
_____HOW TO WRITE A HIT SONG & SELL IT *Tommy Boyce*	7.00
_____JUGGLING MADE EASY *Rudolf Dittrich*	2.00
_____MAGIC MADE EASY *Byron Wels*	2.00
_____SEW SIMPLY, SEW RIGHT *Mini Rhea & F. Leighton*	2.00
_____STAMP COLLECTING FOR BEGINNERS *Burton Hobson*	2.00
_____STAMP COLLECTING FOR FUN & PROFIT *Frank Cetin*	2.00

HORSE PLAYERS' WINNING GUIDES

_____BETTING HORSES TO WIN *Les Conklin*	2.00
_____ELIMINATE THE LOSERS *Bob McKnight*	2.00
_____HOW TO PICK WINNING HORSES *Bob McKnight*	2.00
_____HOW TO WIN AT THE RACES *Sam (The Genius) Lewin*	2.00
_____HOW YOU CAN BEAT THE RACES *Jack Kavanagh*	2.00
_____MAKING MONEY AT THE RACES *David Barr*	2.00
_____PAYDAY AT THE RACES *Les Conklin*	2.00
_____SMART HANDICAPPING MADE EASY *William Bauman*	2.00

HUMOR

_____BILL BALLANCE HANDBOOK OF NIFTY MOVES *Bill Ballance*	3.00
_____HOW TO BE A COMEDIAN FOR FUN & PROFIT *King & Laufer*	2.00

HYPNOTISM

_____ADVANCED TECHNIQUES OF HYPNOSIS *Melvin Powers*	1.00
_____CHILDBIRTH WITH HYPNOSIS *William S. Kroger, M.D.*	2.00
_____HOW TO SOLVE YOUR SEX PROBLEMS	
WITH SELF-HYPNOSIS *Frank S. Caprio, M.D.*	2.00
_____HOW TO STOP SMOKING THRU SELF-HYPNOSIS *Leslie M. LeCron*	2.00
_____HOW TO USE AUTO-SUGGESTION EFFECTIVELY *John Duckworth*	2.00
_____HOW YOU CAN BOWL BETTER USING SELF-HYPNOSIS *Jack Heise*	2.00
_____HOW YOU CAN PLAY BETTER GOLF USING SELF-HYPNOSIS *Heise*	2.00

_____HYPNOSIS AND SELF-HYPNOSIS Bernard Hollander, M.D. 2.00
_____HYPNOTISM (Originally published in 1893) Carl Sextus 3.00
_____HYPNOTISM & PSYCHIC PHENOMENA Simeon Edmunds 2.00
_____HYPNOTISM MADE EASY Dr. Ralph Winn 2.00
_____HYPNOTISM MADE PRACTICAL Louis Orton 2.00
_____HYPNOTISM REVEALED Melvin Powers 1.00
_____HYPNOTISM TODAY Leslie LeCron & Jean Bordeaux, Ph.D. 2.00
_____MODERN HYPNOSIS Lesley Kuhn & Salvatore Russo, Ph.D. 3.00
_____NEW CONCEPTS OF HYPNOSIS Bernard C. Gindes, M.D. 3.00
_____POST-HYPNOTIC INSTRUCTIONS Arnold Furst 2.00
     How to give post-hypnotic suggestions for therapeutic purposes.
_____PRACTICAL GUIDE TO SELF-HYPNOSIS Melvin Powers 2.00
_____PRACTICAL HYPNOTISM Philip Magonet, M.D. 2.00
_____SECRETS OF HYPNOTISM S. J. Van Pelt, M.D. 3.00
_____SELF-HYPNOSIS Paul Adams 2.00
_____SELF-HYPNOSIS Its Theory, Technique & Application Melvin Powers 2.00
_____SELF-HYPNOSIS A Conditioned-Response Technique Laurance Sparks 3.00
_____THERAPY THROUGH HYPNOSIS edited by Raphael H. Rhodes 3.00

JUDAICA

_____HOW TO LIVE A RICHER & FULLER LIFE Rabbi Edgar F. Magnin 2.00
_____MODERN ISRAEL Lily Edelman 2.00
_____OUR JEWISH HERITAGE Rabbi Alfred Wolf & Joseph Gaer 2.00
_____ROMANCE OF HASSIDISM Jacob S. Minkin 2.50
_____SERVICE OF THE HEART Evelyn Garfield, Ph.D. 3.00
_____STORY OF ISRAEL IN COINS Jean & Maurice Gould 2.00
_____STORY OF ISRAEL IN STAMPS Maxim & Gabriel Shamir 1.00
_____TONGUE OF THE PROPHETS Robert St. John 3.00
_____TREASURY OF COMFORT edited by Rabbi Sidney Greenberg 3.00

MARRIAGE, SEX & PARENTHOOD

_____ABILITY TO LOVE Dr. Allan Fromme 3.00
_____ENCYCLOPEDIA OF MODERN SEX & LOVE TECHNIQUES Macandrew 3.00
_____GUIDE TO SUCCESSFUL MARRIAGE Drs. Albert Ellis & Robert Harper 3.00
_____HOW TO RAISE AN EMOTIONALLY HEALTHY, HAPPY CHILD, A. Ellis 2.00
_____IMPOTENCE & FRIGIDITY Edwin W. Hirsch, M.D. 3.00
_____NEW APPROACHES TO SEX IN MARRIAGE John E. Eichenlaub, M.D. 2.00
_____SEX WITHOUT GUILT Albert Ellis, Ph.D. 2.00
_____SEXUALLY ADEQUATE FEMALE Frank S. Caprio, M.D. 2.00
_____SEXUALLY ADEQUATE MALE Frank S. Caprio, M.D. 2.00
_____YOUR FIRST YEAR OF MARRIAGE Dr. Tom McGinnis 2.00

METAPHYSICS & OCCULT

_____BOOK OF TALISMANS, AMULETS & ZODIACAL GEMS William Pavitt 3.00
_____CONCENTRATION—A Guide to Mental Mastery Mouni Sadhu 3.00
_____DREAMS & OMENS REVEALED Fred Gettings 2.00
_____EXTRASENSORY PERCEPTION Simeon Edmunds 2.00
_____FORTUNE TELLING WITH CARDS P. Foli 2.00
_____HANDWRITING ANALYSIS MADE EASY John Marley 2.00
_____HANDWRITING TELLS Nadya Olyanova 3.00
_____HOW TO UNDERSTAND YOUR DREAMS Geoffrey A. Dudley 2.00
_____ILLUSTRATED YOGA William Zorn 2.00
_____IN DAYS OF GREAT PEACE Mouni Sadhu 2.00
_____KING SOLOMON'S TEMPLE IN THE MASONIC TRADITION Alex Horne 5.00
_____MAGICIAN — His training and work W. E. Butler 2.00
_____MEDITATION Mouni Sadhu 3.00
_____MODERN NUMEROLOGY Morris C. Goodman 2.00
_____NUMEROLOGY—ITS FACTS AND SECRETS Ariel Yvon Taylor 2.00
_____PALMISTRY MADE EASY Fred Gettings 2.00
_____PALMISTRY MADE PRACTICAL Elizabeth Daniels Squire 3.00
_____PALMISTRY SECRETS REVEALED Henry Frith 2.00
_____PRACTICAL YOGA Ernest Wood 3.00
_____PROPHECY IN OUR TIME Martin Ebon 2.50

_____ PSYCHOLOGY OF HANDWRITING *Nadya Olyanova*	2.00
_____ SEEING INTO THE FUTURE *Harvey Day*	2.00
_____ SUPERSTITION — Are you superstitious? *Eric Maple*	2.00
_____ TAROT *Mouni Sadhu*	4.00
_____ TAROT OF THE BOHEMIANS *Papus*	3.00
_____ TEST YOUR ESP *Martin Ebon*	2.00
_____ WAYS TO SELF-REALIZATION *Mouni Sadhu*	2.00
_____ WITCHCRAFT, MAGIC & OCCULTISM—A Fascinating History *W. B. Crow*	3.00
_____ WITCHCRAFT — THE SIXTH SENSE *Justine Glass*	2.00
_____ WORLD OF PSYCHIC RESEARCH *Hereward Carrington*	2.00
_____ YOU CAN ANALYZE HANDWRITING *Robert Holder*	2.00

SELF-HELP & INSPIRATIONAL

_____ CYBERNETICS WITHIN US *Y. Saparina*	3.00
_____ DAILY POWER FOR JOYFUL LIVING *Dr. Donald Curtis*	2.00
_____ DOCTOR PSYCHO-CYBERNETICS *Maxwell Maltz, M.D.*	3.00
_____ DYNAMIC THINKING *Melvin Powers*	1.00
_____ GREATEST POWER IN THE UNIVERSE *U. S. Andersen*	4.00
_____ GROW RICH WHILE YOU SLEEP *Ben Sweetland*	2.00
_____ GROWTH THROUGH REASON *Albert Ellis, Ph.D.*	3.00
_____ GUIDE TO DEVELOPING YOUR POTENTIAL *Herbert A. Otto, Ph.D.*	3.00
_____ GUIDE TO LIVING IN BALANCE *Frank S. Caprio, M.D.*	2.00
_____ GUIDE TO RATIONAL LIVING *Albert Ellis, Ph.D. & R. Harper, Ph.D.*	3.00
_____ HELPING YOURSELF WITH APPLIED PSYCHOLOGY *R. Henderson*	2.00
_____ HELPING YOURSELF WITH PSYCHIATRY *Frank S. Caprio, M.D.*	2.00
_____ HOW TO ATTRACT GOOD LUCK *A. H. Z. Carr*	2.00
_____ HOW TO CONTROL YOUR DESTINY *Norvell*	2.00
_____ HOW TO DEVELOP A WINNING PERSONALITY *Martin Panzer*	3.00
_____ HOW TO DEVELOP AN EXCEPTIONAL MEMORY *Young & Gibson*	3.00
_____ HOW TO OVERCOME YOUR FEARS *M. P. Leahy, M.D.*	2.00
_____ HOW YOU CAN HAVE CONFIDENCE AND POWER *Les Giblin*	2.00
_____ HUMAN PROBLEMS & HOW TO SOLVE THEM *Dr. Donald Curtis*	2.00
_____ I CAN *Ben Sweetland*	3.00
_____ I WILL *Ben Sweetland*	2.00
_____ LEFT-HANDED PEOPLE *Michael Barsley*	3.00
_____ MAGIC IN YOUR MIND *U. S. Andersen*	3.00
_____ MAGIC OF THINKING BIG *Dr. David J. Schwartz*	2.00
_____ MAGIC POWER OF YOUR MIND *Walter M. Germain*	3.00
_____ MENTAL POWER THRU SLEEP SUGGESTION *Melvin Powers*	1.00
_____ ORIENTAL SECRETS OF GRACEFUL LIVING *Boye De Mente*	1.00
_____ OUR TROUBLED SELVES *Dr. Allan Fromme*	3.00
_____ PRACTICAL GUIDE TO SUCCESS & POPULARITY *C. W. Bailey*	2.00
_____ PSYCHO-CYBERNETICS *Maxwell Maltz, M.D.*	2.00
_____ SCIENCE OF MIND IN DAILY LIVING *Dr. Donald Curtis*	2.00
_____ SECRET OF SECRETS *U. S. Andersen*	3.00
_____ STUTTERING AND WHAT YOU CAN DO ABOUT IT *W. Johnson, Ph.D.*	2.00
_____ SUCCESS-CYBERNETICS *U. S. Andersen*	3.00
_____ 10 DAYS TO A GREAT NEW LIFE *William E. Edwards*	2.00
_____ THINK AND GROW RICH *Napoleon Hill*	3.00
_____ THREE MAGIC WORDS *U. S. Andersen*	3.00
_____ TREASURY OF THE ART OF LIVING *Sidney S. Greenberg*	3.00
_____ YOU ARE NOT THE TARGET *Laura Huxley*	3.00
_____ YOUR SUBCONSCIOUS POWER *Charles M. Simmons*	3.00
_____ YOUR THOUGHTS CAN CHANGE YOUR LIFE *Dr. Donald Curtis*	2.00

The books listed above can be obtained from your book dealer or directly from Melvin Powers. When ordering, please remit 25c per book postage & handling. Send 25c for our illustrated catalog of self-improvement books.

Melvin Powers

12015 Sherman Road, No. Hollywood, California 91605